Superantigens:
A Pathogen's View
of the Immune System

SERIES EDITORS
John Inglis and Jan A. Witkowski
Cold Spring Harbor Laboratory

CURRENT COMMUNICATIONS
In Cell & Molecular Biology

1 *Electrophoresis of Large DNA Molecules: Theory and Applications*
2 *Cellular and Molecular Aspects of Fiber Carcinogenesis*
3 *Apoptosis: The Molecular Basis of Cell Death*
4 *Animal Applications of Research in Mammalian Development*
5 *Molecular Biology of Free Radical Scavenging Systems*
6 *Lyme Disease: Molecular and Immunologic Approaches*
7 *Superantigens: A Pathogen's View of the Immune System*

CURRENT COMMUNICATIONS 7
In Cell & Molecular Biology

Superantigens:
A Pathogen's View
of the Immune System

Edited by

Brigitte T. Huber
Tufts University

Ed Palmer
Basel Institute for Immunology

Cold Spring Harbor Laboratory Press 1993

CURRENT COMMUNICATIONS 7
In Cell & Molecular Biology
Superantigens: A Pathogen's View of the Immune System

Front Cover: Model of the predicted tri-molecular complex formed by the MHC class II molecule, the superantigen SEA, and the TCR. The model is based on the crystal structures of HLA-A2 and SEB. The TCR-binding site is shown as a depression in the top of the toxin molecule. (Courtesy of J.D. Fraser et al.; see related article by Fraser et al., this volume.)

Back Cover: Model depicting the major differences between a conventional peptide antigen and a superantigen: Superantigens are not processed into peptides and associate with the class II molecule outside the peptide binding groove, probably mainly through the β chain. In addition, superantigen recognition by the TCR is restricted to HVR 4 on the outside of the Vβ chain, whereas the HVR 3 of the combined Vα and Vβ chains is exclusively used for peptide recognition in the context of the MHC class II molecule. (Courtesy of D. Yasui and B.T. Huber, Department of Pathology, Tufts University School of Medicine, Boston.)

Library of Congress Cataloging-in-Publication Data

Superantigens: a pathogen's view of the immune system / edited by
    Brigitte T. Huber, Ed Palmer.
        p. cm. -- (Current communications in cell & molecular biology
    ; 7)
        Includes bibliographical references and index.
        ISBN 0-87969-398-3
        1. Superantigens. I. Huber, Brigitte T.   II. Palmer, Ed. 1952-
        III. Series.
        [DNLM: 1. Antigens, Bacterial--immunology. 2. Antigens, Viral-
    -immunology.   3. T-Lymphocytes--immunology.   4. T-Lymphocytes-
    -physiology.   5. Enterotoxins--immunology.   W1 CU7871 v. 7 1993 /
    QW 573 S9593 1993]
    QR186.6.S94S87   1993
    616.07'92--dc20
    DNLM/DLC
    for Library of Congress   93-37215
                                                                        CIP

All Cold Spring Harbor Laboratory Press publications may be ordered directly from Cold Spring Harbor Laboratory Press, 10 Skyline Drive, Plainview, New York 11803. Phone 1-800-843-4388 (in Continental U.S. and Canada). All other locations: (516) 349-1930. FAX: (516) 349-1946.

Contents

Preface, *vii*

Introduction *1*
B.T. Huber and E. Palmer

Structural Model of Staphylococcal Enterotoxin A Interaction with MHC Class II Antigens *7*
J.D. Fraser, S. Lowe, M.J. Irwin, N.R.J. Gascoigne, and K.R. Hudson

Superantigens Expressed by Mouse Mammary Tumor Virus *31*
H. Acha-Orbea

Superantigen Function in Mouse Mammary Tumor Virus-induced Tumorigenesis *45*
S.R. Ross, T.V. Golovkina, and A. Chervonsky

Polymorphism of TCR Vβ Regions and Clonal Deletions in Wild Mouse Populations *59*
P.N. Marche, E. Jouvin-Marche, and P.-A. Cazenave

T-Cell Recognition of Superantigen: Role of Non-Vβ TCR Elements and MHC Molecules *75*
M.A. Blackman, H.P. Smith, R. Wen, A.M. Deckhut, and D.L. Woodland

MTV-encoded Superantigen Expression in B Lymphoma Cells in SJL Mice as a Stimulus for "Reversed Immunological Surveillance" *93*
V.K. Tsiagbe, J. Asakawa, T. Yoshimoto, S.Y. Cho, D. Meruelo, and G.J. Thorbecke

Superantigenicity of Rabies Virus Nucleocapsid in Humans and Mice   117
M. Lafon, D. Scott-Algara, E. Jouvin-Marche, and P.N. Marche

Superantigens and the Pathogenesis of Viral Diseases   139
H. Soudeyns, N. Rebai, G.P. Pantaleo, F. Denis, A.S. Fauci, and R.-P. Sékaly

HIV-1 Replication in T Cells Dependent on TCR Vβ Expression   163
D.N. Posnett, S. Kabak, A. Asch, and A.S. Hodtsev

Index, 179

Preface

During the past few years, a series of microbial agents have been defined which have a profound effect on the immune system. They are very potent activators of T lymphocytes, similar to mitogens. However, unlike mitogens, these microbial products are specifically recognized by the immune system, causing in vivo deletion and in vitro proliferation of T cells. Thus, the term "superantigen" was coined.

The superantigen character of bacterial toxins has been well studied by many research groups. In addition, the murine mammary tumor virus, a retrovirus, expresses a superantigen. Although superantigens are the causative agents for the deleterious effects of the bacterial toxins, their biological significance for the life cycle of the bacteria is still obscure. On the other hand, evidence has been accumulated that superantigens are an essential component for the transmission of the infectious mammary tumor virus. It has also been suggested that the human immunodeficiency virus, HIV-1, makes use of a superantigen for facilitating viral replication, but the actual gene product has not yet been defined. In addition, the nuclear capsid antigen of rabies virus, a negative-strand RNA virus, behaves as a superantigen.

Superantigens differ in three respects from conventional antigens. First of all, they are not processed into peptides and associate with the major histocompatibility complex (MHC) class II molecules outside the polymorphic peptide-binding groove. Second, although they require MHC class II molecules for presentation, the T-cell response is not MHC-restricted, and superantigens can be presented across species barriers. Finally, superantigens interact with the T-cell receptor over the Vβ segment only, regardless of third hypervariable regions and Vα expression.

In the autumn of 1992, a meeting was convened at the Banbury Center that brought together virologists, biochemists, cellular immunologists, molecular biologists, and crystallographers to discuss the topic of superantigens. Many new insights were gained.

This book is not the proceedings of the meeting. Instead, the discussions there provided a framework for the assembly of a book intended to provide an overview of the immunological intricacies of superantigens to cell biologists, biochemists, and physiologists. It will also serve as a source of detailed information on the various structural and functional aspects of superantigens for the immunologists. Specifically, this book is of value to any graduate student or postdoctoral fellow in biomedical sciences, because it presents in a concise way the definition and functional profile of superantigens.

Special thanks to John Inglis and Jan Witkowskl for editing this series of science books, to the Banbury staff for their help in organizing the meeting, and to the staff of Cold Spring Harbor Laboratory Press, especially Patricia Barker, technical editor, and Inez Sialiano, editorial assistant.

B.T.H
E.P.

Corporate Sponsors

The meetings' programs at Cold Spring Harbor Laboratory are supported by:

Akzo Pharma International B.V.
Alafi Capital Company
American Cyanamid Company
Amgen Inc.
Applied Biosystems, Inc.
Armstrong Pharmaceuticals Inc.
BASF Bioresearch Corporation
Becton Dickinson and Company
Boehringer Mannheim Corporation
Ciba-Geigy Corporation/Ciba-Geigy Limited
Diagnostic Products Corporation
The Du Pont Merck Pharmaceutical Company
Eastman Kodak Company
Genentech, Inc.
Glaxo
Hoffmann-La Roche Inc.
Johnson & Johnson
Kyowa Hakko Kogyo Co., Ltd.
Life Technologies, Inc.
Eli Lilly and Company
MetPath Inc.
Millipore Corporation
Monsanto Company
New England BioLabs, Inc.
Oncogene Science, Inc.
Pall Corporation
Perkin-Elmer Cetus Instruments
Pfizer Inc.
Recordati
Sandoz Research Institute
Schering-Plough Corporation
SmithKline Beecham Pharmaceuticals
Sumitomo Pharmaceuticals Co., Ltd.
Takeda Chemical Industries, Ltd.
Toyobo Co., Ltd.
The Upjohn Company
The Wellcome Research Laboratories,
   Burroughs Wellcome Co.
Wyeth-Ayerst Research

Introduction

B.T. Huber[1] and E. Palmer[2]
[1]Department of Pathology
Tufts University School of Medicine
Boston, Massachusetts 02111
[2]Basel Institute for Immunology
CH-4005 Basel, Switzerland

A Brief History of Superantigens (1973–1993)

Superantigens have occupied the attention of immunologists since 1973, when Festenstein (1973) described unmapped genetic loci encoding antigens that generated vigorous mixed leukocyte reactions (MLRs) between major histocompatibility complex (MHC)-identical strains of mice. The responding cells in these MLRs were T lymphocytes, and the stimulating cells were B lymphocytes. Since these antigenic loci mapped outside the MHC, they were named minor lymphocyte stimulating or Mls antigens. The designation of "minor" was a bit of a misnomer, since it only reflects the fact that the Mls antigens were described after the MHC antigens and ignores the extremely high precursor frequency of Mls-reactive T cells. Among the laboratories working on the Mls antigens, several acronyms were invented to fit the initials M.L.S. One of our favorites was Major/minor League Stuff.

Whereas the MLR represented a striking experimental result, the actual function of MHC and Mls antigens had to be something more important than the amusement of a few immunologists. With time, the role of the MHC-encoded proteins became apparent. The observation that the recognition of foreign antigens by T lymphocytes is "restricted" by the MHC proteins of the responding individual, and that this restriction is the result of a selective process occurring intrathymically during ontogeny, represents a major advance in our understanding of T-cell function. More recent work has shown that foreign proteins are processed (degraded) and the peptide products of processed antigens bind to newly synthesized MHC molecules within the cell. Complexes of foreign peptide and self-MHC

Superantigens: A Pathogen's View of the Immune System
© 1993 Cold Spring Harbor Laboratory Press 0-87969-398-3/93 $5 + .00

proteins are transported to the cell surface to form the actual ligand recognized by the T-cell receptor (TCR). Thus, the function of MHC proteins is to trap foreign peptides intracellularly and to display them to a responding T lymphocyte.

On the other hand, it took longer for the function of the Mls antigens to become apparent. Their intimate relationship with the TCR became clear in 1988 when Kappler, Marrack, and their colleagues (Kappler et al. 1988) and MacDonald et al. (1988) simultaneously described the deletion of T-cell subsets from mice expressing the Mls antigens. Strikingly, these T-cell subsets were defined by the Vβ domain of the TCR. Thus, the Mls antigens are clearly recognized by the TCR, and the major determinant of Mls reactivity is the expression of a particular Vβ domain. This latter property distinguishes the Mls antigens from peptide antigens, in that the recognition of a specific peptide/MHC complex is generally dependent on the structure of the entire TCR, composed of its Vα, Jα, Vβ, Dβ, Nβ, and Jβ components. Furthermore, the Mls antigens are recognized as self-antigens, since Mls-reactive T cells are deleted from the repertoire during ontogeny.

An interesting twist to the superantigen story was the discovery that staphylococcal enterotoxins, secreted proteins that cause food poisoning in humans, have properties similar to the Mls antigens (Janeway et al. 1989; White et al. 1989). Their recognition by a high frequency of T cells is determined by the expression of a particular set of Vβ domains. The Mls antigens and enterotoxins were eventually put under the appellation of superantigens. Perhaps this name is more evocative of the potent mitogenic effects of these proteins. At the time, it seemed puzzling how proteins derived from pathogenic bacteria could have such similar properties to the endogenous Mls antigens of mice. Part of the answer to this dilemma came in 1991, when four laboratories established a genetic linkage between expression of the Mls antigens and the presence of particular endogenous (or infectious) mouse mammary tumor viruses (MMTVs) (Dyson et al. 1991; Frankel et al. 1991; Marrack et al. 1991; Woodland et al. 1991). Additional work showed that the viral superantigen is encoded by an open reading frame encoded within the 3′ long terminal repeat of the virus (Acha-Orbea et al. 1991; Choi et al. 1991). By establishing the molecular identity of the Mls antigens, one of the puzzles of superantigens had been solved; both the endogenous Mls antigens and the exogenous staphylococcal enterotoxins are derived from infectious sources.

Superantigen Function: A 1993 Perspective

Superantigens clearly have profound effects on T lymphocytes. By interacting with T cells through the Vβ domain of the TCR, these proteins are able to activate mature T cells and delete immature thymocytes. For the immunologist, superantigens represent useful reagents to probe the TCR:MHC interaction, although it remains to be shown whether T-cell recognition of a superantigen is fundamentally similar to the recognition of a peptide antigen. Despite the existence of an ample experimental literature describing the rules of TCR:superantigen interactions, one can still legitimately ask, "What do these proteins actually do?" and "Why have they evolved to have MHC- and TCR-binding properties?" Part of the difficulty in addressing these issues comes from the fact that the Mls phenomena have traditionally been viewed from the perspective of the mouse. By analogy with the MHC proteins, it was assumed that Mls genes embedded within the mouse genome would encode proteins required for the proper functioning of the immune system. The discovery that the Mls antigens are derived from mouse mammary tumor proviruses revealed the Mls antigens for what they are, i.e., the products of recently acquired viral genes. It is clear that the Mls antigens did not evolve in a mouse genome but instead in a retroviral genome, and inevitably, one is forced to ask, "What are these antigens doing for the virus?" There may be no simple answer to this question, but recent work from the laboratories of H. Acha-Orbea and H.R. MacDonald (Held et al. 1993) demonstrates a requirement for superantigen expression during MMTV infection. Thus, this class of viruses may have evolved a protein with MHC- and TCR-binding properties to play an important role during infection.

The papers collected in this volume represent the recent transition in thinking about superantigen function. The importance of superantigens as a special class of mitogen/antigen that reveal so much about T-cell development and function cannot be underestimated. However, it seems likely that future work in the field will focus on the potential role played by these proteins as mediators of infectivity.

REFERENCES

Acha-Orbea, H., A.N. Shakhov, L. Scarpellino, E. Kolb, V. Müller, A. Vessaz-Shaw, R. Fuchs, K. Blöchlinger, P. Rollini, J. Billote, M. Sarafidou, H.R. MacDonald, and H. Diggelmann. 1991. Clonal deletion of $V_\beta 14$ positive T cells in mammary tumor virus transgenic mice. *Nature* **350**: 207.

Choi, Y., J.W. Kappler, and P. Marrack. 1991. A superantigen encoded in the open reading frame of the 3' long terminal repeat of mouse mammary tumor virus. *Nature* **350**: 203.

Dyson, P.J., A.M. Knight, S. Fairchild, E. Simpson, and K. Tomonari. 1991. Genes encoding ligands for deletion of $V\beta 11$ T cells cosegregate with mammary tumor virus genomes. *Nature* **349**: 531.

Festenstein, H. 1973. Immunogenetic and biological aspects of in vitro lymphocyte allo-transformation (MLR) in the mouse. *Transplant Rev.* **15**: 62.

Frankel, W.N., C. Rudy, J.M. Coffin, and B.T. Huber. 1991. Linkage of *Mls* genes to endogenous mammary tumor viruses of inbred mice. *Nature* **349**: 526.

Held, W., G.A. Waanders, A.N. Shakov, L. Scarpellino, H. Acha-Orbea, and H.R. MacDonald. 1993. Superantigen-induced immune stimulation amplifies mouse mammary tumor virus infection and allows virus transmission. *Cell* **74**: 529.

Janeway, C.A., Jr., J. Yagi, P.J. Conrad, M.E. Katz, B. Jones, S. Vroegop, and S. Buxser. 1989. T-cell responses to Mls and to bacterial proteins that mimic its behavior. *Immunol. Rev.* **107**: 61.

Kappler, J.W., U.D. Staerz, J. White, and P.C. Marrack. 1988. Self-tolerance eliminates T cells specific for Mls-modified products of the major histocompatibility complex. *Nature* **332**: 35.

MacDonald, H.R., R. Schneider, R.L. Lees, R.K. Howe, H. Acha-Orbea, H. Festenstein, R.M. Zinkernagel, and H. Hengartner. 1988. T-cell receptor $V\beta$ use predicts reactivity and tolerance to Mls[a]-encoded antigens. *Nature* **332**: 40.

Marrack, P.C., E. Kushnir, and J. Kappler. 1991. A maternally inherited superantigen encoded by a mammary tumor virus. *Nature* **349**: 524.

White, J., A. Herman, A.M. Pullen, R. Kubo, J.W. Kappler, and P. Marrack. 1989. The V_β-specific superantigen staphylococcal enterotoxin B: Stimulation of mature T cells and clonal deletion in neonatal mice. *Cell* **56:** 27.

Woodland, D.L., M.P. Happ, K.J. Gollub, and E. Palmer. 1991. An endogenous retrovirus mediating deletion of αβ T cells? *Nature* **349:** 529.

Structural Model of Staphylococcal Enterotoxin A Interaction with MHC Class II Antigens

J.D. Fraser,[1] S. Lowe,[1] M.J. Irwin,[2] N.R.J. Gascoigne,[2] and K.R. Hudson[1]

[1]Department of Molecular Medicine, School of Medicine, University of Auckland, Auckland, New Zealand
[2]Department of Immunology, The Scripps Research Institute, La Jolla California 92037

INTRODUCTION

The staphylococcal enterotoxins are well known as the agents causing staphylococcal food poisoning, but for many years their mechanism was unknown. In 1970, Peavy described the activation of human peripheral blood T cells by purified enterotoxin B (SEB) and provided the first evidence that their primary target was not the gut but T lymphocytes (Peavy et al. 1970). The enteric response was presumably a means by which primates could rid the body of these toxins before they entered the bloodstream. It took an additional 20 years before immunologists noticed that their activity on T cells was identical to the enigmatic endogenous minor lymphocyte-stimulating (Mls) antigens in mice (Festenstein and Kimura 1988; Janeway et al. 1988, 1989; Marrack and Kappler 1990). Since then the staphylococcal enterotoxins or bacterial *superantigens*, as they are now more commonly known, have become important tools in understanding the nature of T-cell activation and evolution of the T-cell repertoire. Although some of their behavior is understood, their exact mechanism of action is still unclear.

The staphylococcal enterotoxins (SE) and homologous streptococcal pyrogenic exotoxins (SPE) have the ability to bind both major histocompatibility complex (MHC) class II antigens and T-cell receptor (TCR) simultaneously, a situation

Superantigens: A Pathogen's View of the Immune System
© 1993 Cold Spring Harbor Laboratory Press 0-87969-398-3/93 $5 + .00

made even more remarkable by the fact that they share this ability with a number of other quite distinct viral and bacterial proteins (Janeway et al. 1989; Marrack and Kappler 1990). Systemic intoxication by any one of the staphylococcal toxins leads to the activation of up to 20% of all peripheral T cells, and the subsequent massive and uncontrolled release of lymphokines can have fatal consequences. A good example of this is the condition toxic shock syndrome, caused by the superantigen TSST-1. The reason reactivity to these proteins has been retained through evolution is not clear, but perhaps there is also some benefit to retaining that region of the TCR responsible for superantigen recognition which balances out the negative aspects. It is significant that *Staphylococcus aureus* and *Streptococcus pyogenes* are both symbiotic with humans. Up to 70% of the population carry *S. aureus* and *S. pyogenes* at any one time, and most individuals have high titers of neutralizing antibodies to some or all of the bacterial superantigens.

The staphylococcal enterotoxins SEA, SEB, SEC1, SEC2, SEC3, SED, SEE, and the non-enterotoxic toxic shock syndrome toxin TSST are highly stable, single-chain polypeptides (Bergdoll 1983). The relative ease with which they can be produced in *S. aureus* strains and in *Escherichia coli* has ensured rapid progress in defining their structure and function. The following section describes a structure/function analysis of two homologous toxins, SEA and SEE, and the mapping of residues involved in both MHC class II and TCR binding. In conjunction with similar studies performed by Kappler et al. (1992) and the recent X-ray crystallographic structure of SEB (Swaminathan et al. 1992), we present a predictive structure of a toxin/MHC class II complex.

Staphylococcal Toxins Have Two Binding Sites

The staphylococcal enterotoxins have two well-defined biochemical functions. The first is an ability to bind to multiple alleles and isotypes of MHC class II antigens from a variety of species (Fischer et al. 1989; Fraser 1989; Scholl et al. 1989b; Mollick et al. 1989). The second is an ability to activate T cells through the Vβ portion of the TCR instead of the traditional antigen-binding "face" that interacts with MHC and peptide (Janeway et al. 1988; White et al. 1989; Choi et al. 1990; Marrack and Kappler 1990). Thus, all T cells activated by a single toxin share the same TCR Vβ regions but are diverse in both TCR α chain and TCR junctional residues (White et al. 1989; Marrack and Kappler 1990). The region of Vβ responsible for superantigen recognition appears to be a region between residues 70 and 74 in TCR Vβ, which from Wu/Kabat analysis defines a fourth hypervariable region (HV4) separate from the complementarity determining regions CDR1 (residues 24–31) and CDR2 (residues 50–62), predicted to bind to the polymorphic residues along the α helices of MHC class II, and CDR3 (residues 96–105), predicted to bind to peptide residues (Chothia et al. 1988; Claverie et al. 1989; Choi et al. 1990; Jores et al. 1990).

The binding of toxins to MHC class II is readily detectable. For instance, the K_d of SEA binding to HLA-DR1 is 36 nM and of SEE to HLA-DR1 is 125 nM (Fraser 1989; Fraser et al. 1992). In contrast, the interaction between toxins and TCR Vβ is very weak and is only significant after SEA has first bound to MHC class II. Toxins immobilized to a solid support still do not activate T cells in the absence of MHC class II (J.D. Fraser et al., unpubl). This has led to speculation that superantigen activation requires the combination of three separate interactions: (1) TCR to MHC; (2) SEA to MHC; (3) SEA to TCR in order to contribute sufficient change in free energy (ΔG) to induce the necessary activation signal through TCR.

There is some debate over the involvement of the TCR to MHC class II interaction. For example, it has been shown that two soluble murine TCR β-chain proteins still bind to SEA plus MHC class II, even though three of its six CDR regions (i.e., those provided by α chain) are missing (Gascoigne and Ames 1991). Therefore, βCDR1 and βCDR2 residues of the TCR make a much greater contribution than αCDR1 and αCDR2, which seem to be superfluous. Alternatively, the TCR to MHC class II interaction is not required, and the essential role of MHC class II is not to bind TCR but to induce a conformational change in the toxin structure that increases its affinity toward TCR Vβ. Evidence so far predicts that the interaction between the TCR and MHC class II is required in superantigen activation. For instance, Herman et al. (1990) have shown that polymorphisms in MHC class II do affect the response of individual Vβs to a single toxin.

Toxins Bind to Different Regions in the Polymorphic Domains of MHC Class II

Amino acid sequence comparison of all bacterial super-antigens, including the related streptococcal pyrogenic exotoxins SPE-A and SPE-B, indicates that except perhaps for TSST, all have evolved from a single ancestral gene, but the family can be segregated into three distinct groups (Fig. 1). Group 1 contains SEA, SED, and SEE; group 2 contains SEB, SEC1, SEC3, SPE-A, and SPE-C; and group 3 contains only TSST. These groupings are not based solely on primary sequence homology, but also reflect important functional differences in the region of MHC class II to which they bind. For example, competition binding studies with SEA, SEB, and TSST to human B cells expressing HLA-DR antigens indicate three separate but overlapping binding sites. SEA competes equally well with both SEB and TSST (Fraser 1989; Pontzer et al. 1991; Purdie et al. 1991), but SEB and TSST do not compete at all in binding studies (Scholl et al. 1989a; Purdie et al. 1991). Thus, divergence in the bacterial superantigen family appears to have come about through the selection of toxins that bind to slightly different regions of MHC class II. The impact this may have on general TCR activation is discussed more fully below. Several MHC class II residues important for the binding of SEA and TSST have been mapped (Karp et al. 1990; Herman et al. 1991; Russel et al. 1990, 1991; Karp and Long 1992; Panina-Bordignon et al. 1992). Notably, all these residues are in the distal domains of MHC class II close to the region involved with TCR binding, but they map to opposite sides of the MHC class II peptide groove (Brown et al. 1988).

Production of SEA and SEE and SEA/SEE Hybrids from E. coli

One serious limitation of using *S. aureus*-derived toxins is the contamination by one or more toxins from a single bacterial isolate; because of their biochemical similarity, the toxins are

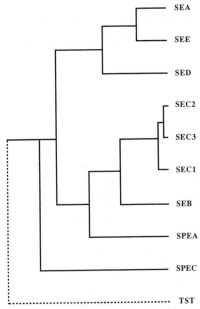

SEA
SEE
SED
SEC2
SEC3
SEC1
SEB
SPEA
SPEC
TST

FIGURE 1 Bacterial superantigen family tree. On the basis of amino acid homology, the toxins can be divided into three functional types. Type I toxins (SEA, SED, and SEE) require zinc to bind to MHC class II, whereas types II and III do not. The MHC class II binding site for type I toxins overlaps with type II and type III, but type II and type II binding sites are distinct.

extremely difficult to separate completely. To circumvent this problem, the genes for SEA and SEE were cloned and expressed in *E. coli*, and under the endogenous staphylococcal promoter, both SEA and SEE were produced in moderate amounts as mature periplasmic proteins. To increase yield and ease of purification, SEA and SEE were produced as a fusion protein with glutathione transferase (GST) under the *lacZ* promoter (Smith and Johnson 1988). Currently, fusion protein is produced in amounts up to 30 mg/l as a soluble intracellular product which is readily purifed by affinity chromatography in a single step from sonicated bacterial lysates on glutathione agarose. The linker region between toxin and GST is highly sensitive to trypsin, so that fusion protein can be quantitatively cleaved by as little as 0.2 μg/ml TPCK trypsin within 10 minutes at 37°C. In this way we have isolated milligram amounts of both wild-type toxins and a large number of mutants and hybrids, all of which fold normally to produce native, highly active toxins (Hudson et al. 1993).

THE TCR BINDING SITE

Determining the hVβ Response to SEA and SEE

The human TCR Vβ repertoire consists of at least 50 different gene segments, some of which are responsive to SEA and SEE. To determine which Vβs respond to SEA, SEE, and other bacterial toxins, we devised a single-tube reverse dot-blot polymerase chain reaction (PCR) technique to characterize the enrichment of 15 different Vβ genes in toxin-activated peripheral blood lymphocyte (PBL) samples (Hudson et al. 1993). In this method, RNA from toxin-stimulated PBL is reverse-transcribed with a Cβ-specific primer. Second strand is synthesized on the TCR β-chain template with two inosine-containing redundant primers that hybridize to a central conserved region within all hVβ genes. The 5′ end of these redundant primers is fully conserved, allowing amplification with a 5′ anchor primer and a downstream Cβ primer. The radiolabeled 500-bp PCR product is then reverse-hybridized to a collection of immobilized Vβ probes bound to nylon strips. The relative proportion of each Vβ is then determined by the intensity of individual spots on the strips. With this method, we have determined the total human Vβ response to SEA and SEE in a number of individuals. SEA enriched hVβ1.1, -5.3, -6.3, -6.4, -6.9, -7.4, -9.1, and -23.1, whereas SEE enriched hVβ5.1, -6.3, -6.4, -6.9, and -8.1. These profiles were invariant among many different individuals who expressed a variety of MHC class II alleles. This technique was used to map those variable residues betweeen SEA and SEE that dictated either the SEA-like or SEE-like Vβ response.

Mapping the Vβ-determining Residues Using SEA/SEE Hybrids

To map the TCR Vβ determinant of SEA and SEE, a panel of hybrids was constructed using two shared restriction sites generating four separate hybrids, AAE, AEE, EEA, and EAA, which divided the toxins into thirds at residues 85 and 156 in the 233-amino acid polypeptides (Fig. 2). AEE and AAE gave identical patterns to SEE, whereas the Vβ responses to EAA and EEA were identical to SEA, indicating that the Vβ de-

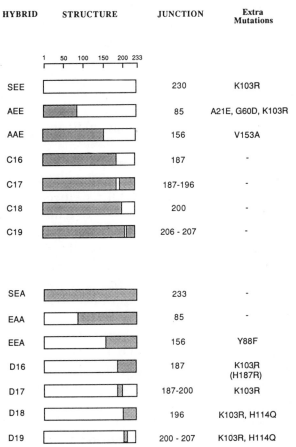

HYBRID	STRUCTURE	JUNCTION	Extra Mutations
SEE		230	K103R
AEE		85	A21E, G60D, K103R
AAE		156	V153A
C16		187	-
C17		187-196	-
C18		200	-
C19		206 - 207	-
SEA		233	-
EAA		85	-
EEA		156	Y88F
D16		187	K103R (H187R)
D17		187-200	K103R
D18		196	K103R, H114Q
D19		200 - 207	K103R, H114Q

FIGURE 2 Structure of SEA/SEE hybrids. Hybrids were constructed by PCR, expressed in *E. coli* as a fusion protein with GST, and purified on GSH agarose. After separation of toxin from GST with trypsin, each hybrid was purified to homogeneity by ion exchange chromatography on CM-Sepharose. Extra mutations were found during sequencing that were introduced by the misincorporation by *Taq* polymerase during PCR. Two versions of D16 have been constructed due to the fact that H187A had a major effect on function.

termining residues were contained within the final 77 carboxy-terminal residues 156–233 (Table 1). This region is relatively invariant between SEA and SEE except for a cluster of variability between residues 187–200 and several isolated regions from 200–233.

To further locate the individual Vβ-determining residues in the carboxy-terminal region, hybrids were constructed with diminishing portions of the carboxy-terminal regions of SEA on SEE (D-series) and vice versa (C-series) (Fig. 2). All hybrids assumed a normal conformation as judged by their ability to activate at similar levels to the parent toxins and their total resistance to trypsin digest. These were tested in the PCR assay to determine the Vβ response profiles. The penultimate hybrids C18 (SEA200SEE) and D18 (SEE196SEA) gave Vβ profiles identical to SEE and SEA, respectively, indicating that Vβ determinant must be located within the final carboxy-terminal 37 amino acids (Table 1). Moreover, the considerable variability in the amino-terminal portion between SEA and SEE contributed little if anything to Vβ specificity. In the last 30 residues there are only 5 variable positions—S/P206, N/D207, M/L224, I/L228, and S/T233 in SEA/SEE; S206P and N207D are nonconservative changes. Two final hybrids, C19 (SEA-P206D207) and D19 (SEE-S206N207), were constructed. Remarkably, switching these residues alone was sufficient to reverse the TCR Vβ profiles between SEA and SEE (Table 1). Only Vβ5.1 and Vβ8.1, which are normally specific for SEE, did not segregate completely with these two residues. Vβ5.1 and Vβ8.1 appeared to be activated by D19 as well as C19, but to a much lesser extent (Hudson et al. 1993). Thus, these two residues were likely candidates for contact residues with TCR Vβ.

To confirm these findings, analysis of all the hybrids was also performed on two T-cell lines. The murine T-cell line SO3 (mVβ17) responded to SEA and D19 (SEE-S206N207) but not to SEE and C19 (SEA-P206D207), whereas Jurkat (hVβ8.1) responded to SEE and SEA-P206D207 but not to SEA. Jurkat was also activated strongly by SEE-S206N207, consistent with the results from the human Vβ profiles indicating that another variable region outside of 206 and 207 influenced Vβ8.1 response (Table 1).

Residues 206 and 207 Determine Direct TCR β-Chain Binding

We have developed a plate binding assay using two soluble murine β-chain proteins mVβ3 and mVβ11, which are secreted from B cells in the absence of any TCR α chain (Gascoigne and Ames 1991). These soluble single-chain TCRs retain the ability to bind cells expressing toxin/MHC class II complexes, indicating that the α chain contributes very little to binding during superantigen recognition. Soluble mVβ3 and mVβ11 readily distinguish SEA and SEE, respectively, but only when toxin is first bound to a human MHC class-II-expressing B cell (Raji). The panel of SEA/SEE hybrids was tested to determine whether residues 206 and 207 also determined β-chain binding. B cells incubated with any of the C-series hybrids including C19 (SEA-P206D207) selectively bound to mVβ11-coated plates and not to mVβ3 plates, whereas B-cells preincubated with any of the D-series hybrids including D19 (SEE-S206N207) selectively bound to mVβ3 (Table 1) (Irwin et al. 1992). Thus residues 206 and 207 were contact points with TCR Vβ and confirmed that the differential response was due to physical contact between residues 206 and 207 and residues within TCR β chain. Residues 206 and 207 are unlikely to be the complete Vβ-binding site, however. These experiments could only pinpoint variable residues in the site. Others such as N25 and Y62 identified by Kappler et al. (1992) were invariant between SEA and SEE.

THE MHC CLASS II BINDING SITE

The Very Amino Terminus of SEA Contributes to MHC Class II Binding

The SEA/SEE hybrids were also informative in identifying regions involved in the MHC class II binding site. The dissociation constant (K_d) for each of the hybrids has been measured using the human B-lymphoblastoid line LG-2 (HLA-DR1,1) (Table 1). SEA binds with a K_d of 36 nM, whereas SEE binds with a K_d of 150 nM. One region that stands out in the analysis of the hybrids is the amino-terminal region. For instance, the AEE hybrid binds with a similar affinity to SEA (K_d = 56

TABLE 1 *FUNCTIONAL DATA FOR THE SEA/SEE HYBRIDS*

Hybrid	Prolif. P_{50} (pg/ml)	MHC binding K_d to DR1 (nM)	hVβ enrichment[a] (>twofold increase)	TCR β-chain binding[b] (cells bound)		Stimulation[c] (IL-2 units/ml)	
				Vβ3	Vβ11	SO3	Jurkat
SEE	3.0	120	5.1,6.3,6.4,6.9,8.1	0	13,000	0	>640
AEE	2.0	56	5.1,6.3,6.4,6.9,8.1	0	5,000	0	>640
AAE	5.0	156	5.1,6.3,6.4,6.9,8.1	0	5,000	0	>640
C16	2.0	75	5.1,6.3,6.4,6.9,8.1	n.d.	n.d.	0	>640
C17	2.0	n.d.	1.1,5.3,6.3,6.4,6.9,7.4,9.1,23.1	n.d.	n.d.	150	0
C18	2.0	36	5.1,6.3,6.4,6.9,8.1	0	11,000	0	>640
C19	2.0	43	5.1,6.3,6.4,6.9,8.1	0	11,000	82	>640

SEA	2.0	36	1.1,5.3,6.3,6.4,6.9,7.4,9.1,23.1	6,000	0	>640	0
EAA	0.5	156	1.1,5.3,6.3,6.4,6.9,7.4,9.1,23.1	15,000	0	>640	80
EEA	2.0	211	1.1,5.3,6.3,6.4,6.9,7.4,9.1,23.1	16,000	0	>640	0
D16	2.0	211	1.1,5.3,6.3,6.4,6.9,7.4,9.1,23.1	n.d.	n.d.	n.d.	n.d.
(D16							
H187A)	66	1440	5.3,6.3,6.4,6.9,7.4,23.1	2,000	0	0	0
D17	1.0	n.d.	5.1,6.3,6.4,6.9,8.1	n.d.	0	0	>640
D18	3.0	720	1.1,5.3,6.3,6.4,6.9,7.4,9.1,23.1	7,000	0	320	>640
D19	0.3	225	1.1,5.1,5.3,6.3,6.4,6.9,7.4,8.1,9.1,23.1	6,000	0	300	>640

All the hybrids were tested for both MHC class II binding and TCR interaction. P_{50} is the concentration required to obtain half-maximal thymidine incorporation in PBL culture. The K_d was determined in a competitive binding assay against ^{125}I SEA to LG-2 cells (homozygous DR1). n.d. indicates not determined.

[a] hVβ enrichment was determined for each hybrid as described previously (Hudson et al. 1993) and those Vβs showing greater than twofold enrichment over resting PBL cultures are given.

[b] TCR β-chain binding was determined as described previously (Gascoigne and Ames 1991). Figures represent the number of class II expressing cells (Raji) bound to the TCR β-chain coated plates in the presence of hybrid toxins.

[c] Two T-cell lines SO3 (mVβ17) and Jurkat (hVβ8.1) were stimulated in the presence of toxin and formalin-fixed LG-2 cells. One unit of IL-2 is the amount required to maintain 50% growth of IL-2-dependent, lectin-activated mouse spleen cells (Hudson et al. 1993).

nM) compared with 156 nM for EAA. This difference in affinity between SEA and SEE can in part be attributed to the very amino-terminal residues. Although identical in sequence, SEE is missing the first three amino acids of SEA. A three-residue truncation variant of SEA at the very amino terminus was constructed and found to have a binding affinity toward HLA-DR1 that was threefold less than SEA. Futhermore, addition of a single glycine residue to the end of SEA results in a threefold reduction in binding affinity (not shown). Thus, the very amino terminus of the toxin influences MHC class II binding, consistent with the results of Pontzer et al. (1989), who have shown that a synthetic peptide to the amino terminus of SEA inhibits MHC class II binding. These findings are relevant when one considers the position of the amino terminus in the crystal structure of SEB. Residues 1 and 2 of SEA lie directly over the zinc atom (Fig. 3).

Zinc Is Required in MHC Class II Binding of SEA, SED, and SEE

Addition of low levels of EDTA completely abolishes SEA, SED, and SEE binding either to MHC class-II-expressing cells or to purified HLA-DR1 (Fraser et al. 1992). The loss of binding in the presence of EDTA is striking and appears to destroy not only specific binding, but also the nonspecific binding of SEA to MHC class-II-expressing B cells (determined by competition of radiolabeled tracer with saturating levels of unlabeled SEA), which is usually about 10% of the specific binding. Reconstitution of binding can only occur when trace amounts of zinc are added in excess over the chelating agent. Strikingly, no other cation so far tested can restore binding except cobalt, which is most similar to zinc and can often substitute in other zinc metalloenzymes without loss of activity (Vallee and Auld 1990). Only the type-1 toxins SEA, SED, and SEE require zinc for binding (Fraser et al. 1992). The binding of both type-2 toxin SEB and type-3 toxin TSST is unaffected by EDTA. The K_d of zinc for SEA has been determined at 1 μM by means of Scatchard analysis, and there is only one zinc atom per SEA molecule.

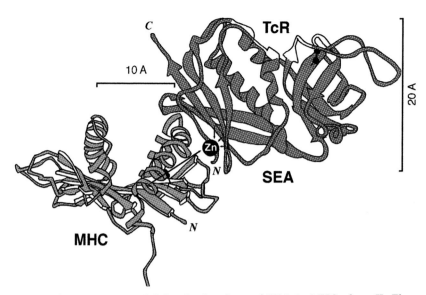

FIGURE 3 Predicted model for the binding of SEA to MHC class II. The model uses the crystal structure of HLA-A2 which is similar to MHC class II (Brown et al. 1988) and the crystal structure of SEB (Swaminathan et al. 1992). The TCR-binding site is clearly shown as a depression in the top of the toxin molecule. The α-carbon atoms of the contact residues S206,N207 are located in the bottom left of this groove. The zinc atom is located on the bottom of the toxin in a region containing H187, H225, and D227, the predicted positions of which are given by arrows. Each side chain is predicted to face to the left of the loop situated beneath the amino-terminal residues. If the zinc site is juxtaposed to H81 in DRβ (arrow) and the toxin is rotated 180° on the horizontal around the zinc atom, the toxin would then bridge the end of the peptide groove, thus interfering with the predicted TSST binding site on the α1 domain. The TCR binding site would point upward and S206,N207 would be situated about 4–5 Å above the MHC α helices in a position amenable to interaction with the HV4 loop of TCR Vβ.

Mapping the Zinc-binding Site in SEA

One hybrid D16 (SEE187SEA) was found in both proliferation studies and cell-binding assays to have reduced activity (Table 1). Sequencing of the D16 gene construct revealed a single mutation H187R inadvertantly introduced by *Taq* polymerase during DNA amplification. Given that this mutation involves a histidine residue, we speculated that it was part of the zinc-binding site because the imidazole nitrogen of histidine is a favored ligand for zinc coordination in all other metalloen-zymes (Vallee and Auld 1990). Other zinc-binding residues used in zinc coordination are cysteine, aspartate, and glu-tamate residues. Two mutants of SEA at this position, SEA-H187R and SEA-H187A, were constructed and tested for proliferation activity, MHC class II binding, and ^{65}Zn binding. The latter assay employed a dot-blot technique whereby EDTA-treated proteins were immobilized to nitrocellulose, then incubated briefly with 1 μM ^{65}ZnCl$_2$. After washing in metal-free buffer, the blots were autoradiographed, and the spots were counted. All mutants at H187 bound between 7-fold and 10-fold less ^{65}Zn than either native SEA, SEE, or SED, and this reflected in their inability to bind to MHC class II and sub-sequently stimulate T cells (Table 2). Interestingly, SED is D187, but this did not affect its ability to bind ^{65}Zn. Thus, position 187 can accommodate a histidine or an aspartic acid but not arginine or alanine. This was strong evidence that position 187 was part of the zinc-binding site. In SEB, the equivalent position is an isoleucine, which may in part explain this toxin's inabilty to bind zinc. Although reduced, zinc bind-ing to the SEA-H187A mutant was not completely destroyed, and increasing the zinc concentration to 7-10 μM allowed the SEA-H187A mutant to bind to MHC class II at 50% of its max-imal binding. Wild-type SEA required 0.7 μM for 50% maximal binding. Thus, the H187A did not alter the MHC class II bind-ing site significantly but reduced its affinity for zinc.

On the basis of a global zinc-binding motif, L1-X$_{(1-3)}$-L2-X$_{(20-40)}$-L3, found in other zinc metalloproteins (Vallee and Auld 1990), we assumed that H187 might be L1 and E191 might be L2 because this residue is conserved in SEA, SEE, and SED. The bidentate structure is globally conserved in all zinc-binding metalloproteins that bind zinc on the surface. In contrast, zinc-finger proteins bind zinc very tightly in a 4-fold coordination with cysteine sulfur atoms in the internal hydrophobic core where the zinc is not accessible to chelating agents or water. In the former class of zinc proteins, the bidentate residues are always spaced one, two, or three residues apart, presumably depending on whether they are on a β strand (one-residue spacing) or an α helix (two- or three-residue spacing). We mutated E191 and all other histidine,

TABLE 2 MAPPING OF ZINC-BINDING RESIDUES IN WILD-TYPE AND MUTANT TOXINS

Mutation	Zinc binding (% of SEA)	MHC binding K_d DR1 (nM)	Proliferation P_{50} (pg/ml)
SEA	100	36	2
SEE	100	120	2
SED	150	n.d.	2
SEB	8	340	10
TSST	<1	130	30
SEA-H187A	14	1440	66
SEA-E191A	100	38	1.0
SEA-E222A	100	36	0.8
SEA-H225A	<1	36,000	1000
SEA-D227A	<1	>50,000	>10,000

All possible zinc-binding amino acids in the carboxyl terminus of H187 were mutated to alanine. To determine zinc binding, mutants were blotted onto nitrocellulose in triplicate and incubated with 1 μM $^{65}ZnCl_2$ for 10 min. After brief washing, spots were cut and counted. Figures represent the relative amount of ^{65}Zn bound as a percentage of wild-type SEA binding. Each purified mutant was also tested for MHC class II binding affinity and T-cell proliferation as described in text.

aspartate, or glutamate residues in the final carboxy-terminal 46 amino acids (there are 6 in total). Mutations E191A and E222A had no effect on either zinc binding, MHC class II binding, or T-cell proliferation. However, mutation H225A reduced MHC class II binding 1000-fold, and D227A obliterated all activity (Table 2). Thus, the zinc-binding site in SEA and SEE is H187.H225.D227, whereas in SED it is D187.H225.D227. This arrangement defines a novel motif because the essential bidentate segment is carboxy-terminal to the L3 ligand. This is opposite to the global zinc-binding motif. Presumably, H225-D227 are on a β strand because they are spaced only one residue apart. Both side chains must point in the same direction out from the protein surface. More importantly, D227 is clearly the most important ligand. This suggests that D225 is itself a bidentate coordination site providing both a carboxylate and a charged hydroxyl group to zinc (this is known to occur infrequently in other zinc metalloproteins). This would require a special environment to ensure the deprotonation of the hydroxyl group at neutral pH.

Zinc Forms a Molecular Bridge with a Residue in MHC Class II

We favor a mechanism whereby zinc actively contributes to the binding energy between toxin and MHC class II. For this to happen, a zinc bridge must be formed between H187.H225.D227 and a residue from MHC class II completing a stable tetravalent coordination complex around zinc. Several recent experiments support this hypothesis. Initial studies showed that addition of purified HLA-DR1 to SEA did not increase the amount of zinc bound (Fraser et al. 1992). This led us to speculate that all the coordination ligands were in SEA and that zinc was required solely for structural purposes (Fraser et al. 1992). However, when the mutant SEA-H187A, which binds ^{65}Zn poorly, was used (Table 2), addition of HLA-DR1 increased the level of ^{65}Zn binding to that of wild-type SEA. Therefore, reducing the toxin component of zinc binding highlights the contribution from MHC class II (K.R. Hudson et al., in prep.). This effect can be explained by viewing the difference in the stability between a 3-fold versus a 4-fold complex as negligible, whereas the difference in stability between 2-fold and 3-fold is major. Thus, zinc appears to contribute a coordination site to a residue in MHC class II. With the displacement of water (which is probably bound to zinc in the free toxin) and the replacement by the MHC class II residue, the zinc coordination complex becomes a stable tetrahedral structure within a hydrophobic interface. This must act as a strong stabilizing force in the toxin/MHC class II complex. Several other experiments suggest that the zinc atom is sandwiched in the hydrophobic interface between MHC class II and SEA and is inaccessible to both water and ionic chelating agents. Initial pH titration experiments showed that SEA/DR1 binding was very sensitive to pH, presumably due to imidazole titration of the zinc-reactive H187 and H225 (pK = 6.5). Only 10% of SEA binding was observed at pH 6.0 and pH 9.0, compared to the maximum at pH 7.5. However, a preformed complex of SEA/DR1 is very stable in the pH range 3–10.5 (J.D. Fraser et al., unpubl.). Moreover, a similar effect has been observed with EDTA, which strips radioactive ^{65}Zn from the interface of a toxin/DR1 complex at a rate 10,000-fold lower than from free SEA. Thus, binding involves the total exclusion of water from the interface, including the water molecule bound to zinc, which we believe is displaced in favor of an MHC class II residue.

The Position of the TCR-binding Site on SEA

The recently resolved crystal structure of SEB (Swaminathan et al. 1992) provides a structure on which to position the two binding sites. Enterotoxins A and B share only 30% identity, but most of the variability falls within regions linking strands and helices, whereas the important structural residues are sufficiently conserved to suggest that both toxins fold into similar structures. The SEB structure consists of two globular domains. The first is formed from residues 29–120. The second and larger domain is formed from residues 121–239 plus 1–29 from the amino terminus. A shallow groove exists between the two domains (Fig. 3). TCR contact residues S206 and N207 identified in SEA and those identified by Kappler et al. (1992), namely N23 and Y61, are all located within this groove. Thus, this region is most likely the TCR Vβ-binding site, which contacts the HV4 domain (residues 70–74) in TCR Vβ.

The Position of the MHC Class II Binding Site on SEA

The zinc-binding site H187.H225.D227 is located at the very bottom of domain 2, approximately 15 Å from the base of the TCR-binding site (Fig. 3). H187 is located on the inner side of a loop, and H225 and D227 are located on a β strand facing H187. All side chains point to the left of the loop structure and are sufficiently close that they form a cluster of residues capable of binding a zinc atom. The amino terminus lies over the top of the zinc site, which is consistent with the results implicating the very amino terminus of SEA in MHC class II binding.

SEA Binds across the End of the Peptide Groove of MHC Class II

His-81 in DRβ1 has been implicated in the SEA-binding site and is essential for binding SEA and SEE but not SEB

(Herman, et al. 1991; Karp and Long 1992). TSST, on the other hand, employs residues M36 and K39 in the DRα1 (Panina-Bordignon et al. 1992). Importantly, both SEA and TSST compete for binding to HLA-DR. Thus, both toxins appear to bind to the end of the peptide groove rather than to the side. One possibility is that H81 in DRβ represents the fourth zinc coordination site. If SEA is placed across the open end of the peptide groove of HLA-DR (facing out of the page in Fig. 3) so that the zinc of SEA is close to H81 in DRβ, the TCR Vβ site would then point upward and the TCR contact residues 206 and 207 of SEA would then be about 4 Å above the MHC class II helices in an ideal position to bind to residues of the HV4 loop in TCR Vβ. Moreover, the TCR CDR1, -2, and -3 regions would still be able to interact with the α helices of MHC class II.

Model of TCR/MHC Interaction

Although no crystal structure of a TCR has been determined, several models have been constructed from immunoglobulin protein folding (Chothia et al. 1988; Davis and Bjorkman 1988; Claverie et al. 1989; Jores et al. 1990). The region of TCR that interacts with superantigens has been shown to be a hypervariable loop in Vβ between residues 70 and 74 (HV4) located to one side of the antigen-binding face (Choi et al. 1990; Pontzer et al. 1992). The crest of the HV4 loop lies on the same plane as the antigen-binding face but to one side of the βCDR1 and βCDR2 loops (Claverie et al. 1989; Jores et al. 1990).

A model has been proposed by Davis and Bjorkman (1988) which predicts that TCR is oriented on MHC in such a way that the Vβ HV4 loop would overhang one side of an MHC α helix. This model is favored because of the relative distances of the CDR regions of both TCR chains, and the position of αCDR3 and βCDR3 fits very well with the dimensions of the known three-dimensional structure of MHC class I. One problem with this model, however, is that each TCR chain must contact only one MHC α helix, which would predict a strong correlation between Vβ expression and MHC haplotype in vivo, a situation that has been found not to occur. To counter this, Davis and Bjorkman suggest that TCR may freely bind to MHC in a 180° rotational orientation and also in different registers along the α helices.

It is also possible to rotate the TCR 90° around the vertical axis on MHC. In this case, each TCR chain would contact both MHC α helices, and the TCR HV4 loop would reside at one end of the peptide groove. One reason that this second model is not favored is that the CDR3s of both chains are forced to lie over the center of the peptide groove, thus limiting their interaction to the very middle of the peptide. However, this is less of a problem when considering recent X-ray crystallographic evidence from a single peptide bound within MHC class I. These structures show that the ends of the peptide are buried deep within the groove inaccessible to TCR, and only the very center of the peptide kinks upward and out of the groove. Side chains from these residues would extend far enough above the MHC α helices to allow interaction with TCR (Madden et al. 1991; Fremont et al. 1992).

Our current knowledge of toxin binding allows us to predict the nature of TCR/MHC interactions because binding to both MHC class II and TCR is asymmetric. Thus, all TCRs expressing a particular Vβ must be oriented on MHC class II in exactly the same way to ligate to toxin, discounting the idea that TCR can bind to MHC class II in different orientations and registers. Second, if toxins do bind at one end of the peptide groove instead of to the side, then the TCR HV4 loop must also lie over the end in order to contact toxin. Thus, superantigen binding favors the second model of TCR/MHC interaction where each TCR chain interacts with both MHC α helices. Some Vβs, by nature of the overall folding, may lie in a slightly different position relative to MHC class II. This would help to explain why three distinct binding sites on MHC class II for type 1, 2, and 3 toxins have evolved. For instance, SED stimulates roughly the same group of Vβs as both SEA and SEE (all type 1 toxins) even though its TCR-binding site is less like SEA and SEE than SEB, which reacts with a completely different set of Vβs. It appears that although variation in the TCR-binding site accounts for some of the differences in Vβ specificity, there is also a correlation between Vβ reactivity and the position of the toxin on MHC class II. We have attempted to convert the TCR-binding site of SEA into SEB by exchanging those residues predicted to be TCR contact residues. Surprisingly, the Vβ stimulation profile of this new mutant does not change significantly toward an SEB profile (J.D. Fraser et al., unpubl), providing further evidence for this hypothesis.

SUMMARY

Although the exact nature of superantigen binding to MHC class II and TCR must await a crystal structure of a toxin/MHC class II complex, much insight can still be obtained from current information, such as the likely binding site on MHC class II and the orientation of toxins in relation to TCR, as we have provided in this paper. It remains to be seen whether other superantigens such as those encoded by the MMTV retrovirus also interact with MHC class II in the same way. Many aspects of superantigen activation remain a complete puzzle. For instance, how and why have such widely divergent proteins as the MMTV and bacterial superantigens converged on a complex biological activity involving the simultaneous binding to two highly polymorphic proteins such as MHC class II and TCR? By nature, it would seem a relatively simple task for TCRs to mutate the HV4 region of Vβ so that it no longer interacted with these toxins—unless the HV4 region has an essential role in T-cell recognition or development so that it cannot be dispensed with. It is somewhat surprising that there are not many more examples of superantigens throughout nature than those found in a few bacteria and viruses, given the apparent diversity of the currently known superantigens.

Superantigens have enriched our knowledge of the T-cell immune system and its evolution in response to a number of microbial pathogens. They will continue to be used as powerful tools in the study of T-cell activation, tolerance, and in vivo deletion. Whether other superantigens will be found, including those for MHC class I, remains to be seen.

ACKNOWLEDGMENTS

The authors gratefully acknowledge the support of the Health Research Council of New Zealand, the Auckland Medical Research Foundation, and the National Institutes of Health Concern Foundation for Cancer Research. J.D.F. is a fellow of the Wellcome Trust (U.K.) and N.R.J.G. is a fellow of the Leukemia Society of America.

REFERENCES

Bergdoll, M.S. 1983. The enterotoxins. In *Staphylococcal and streptococcal infections* (ed. C.S.F. Easom and C. Aslam), p. 559. Academic Press, New York.

Brown, J.H., T. Jardetzky, M.A. Saper, B. Samraoui, P.J. Bjorkman, and D.C. Wiley. 1988. A hypothetical model of the foreign antigen binding site of class II histocompatibility molecules. *Nature* **332:** 845.

Choi, Y.W., A. Herman, D. DiGiusto, T. Wade, P. Marrack, and J. Kappler. 1990. Residues of the variable region of the T-cell-receptor beta-chain that interact with *S. aureus* toxin superantigens. *Nature* **346:** 471.

Chothia, C., D.R. Boswell, and A.M. Lesk. 1988. The outline structure of the T-cell $\alpha\beta$ receptor. *EMBO J.* **7:** 3745.

Claverie. J.-M., A. Prochnicka-Chalufour, and L. Bourgeleret. 1989. Implications of a Fab-like structure for the T-cell receptor. *Immunol. Today* **10:** 10.

Davis, M.M. and P.J. Bjorkman. 1988. T-cell antigen receptor genes and T-cell recognition. *Nature* **334:** 395.

Festenstein, H. and S. Kimura. 1988. The Mls system: Past and present. *J Immunogenet.* **15:** 183.

Fischer, H., M. Dohlsten, M. Lindvall, H. Sjogren, and R. Carlsson. 1989. Binding of staphylococcal enterotoxin A to HLA-DR on B cell lines. *J. Immunol.* **142:** 3151.

Fraser, J.D. 1989. High-affinity binding of staphylococcal enterotoxins A and B to HLA-DR. *Nature* **339:** 221.

Fraser, J.D., R.G. Urban, J.L. Strominger, and H. Robinson. 1992. Zinc regulates the function of two superantigens. *Proc. Natl. Acad. Sci..* **89:** 5507.

Fremont, D.H., M. Matsumura, E.A. Stura, P.A. Peterson, and I.A. Wilson. 1992. Crystal structures of 2 viral peptides in complex with murine MHC class-I H-2K(b). *Science* **257:** 919.

Gascoigne, N.R.J. and C.T. Ames. 1991. Direct binding of secreted T-cell receptor β-chain to superantigen associated with class II major histocompatibility complex protein. *Proc. Natl. Acad. Sci.* **88:** 613.

Herman, A., G. Croteau, R.-P. Sékaly, J. Kappler, and P. Marrack. 1990. HLA-DR alleles differ in their ability to present staphylococcal enterotoxins to T cells. *J. Exp. Med.* **172:** 709.

Herman, A., N. Labrecque, J. Thibodeau, P. Marrack, J.W. Kappler, and R.-P. Sékaly. 1991. Identification of the staphylococcal enterotoxin A superantigen binding site in the beta 1 domain of the human histocompatibility antigen HLA-DR. *Proc. Natl. Acad. Sci.* **88:** 9954.

Hudson, K.R., H. Robinson, and J.D. Fraser. 1993. Two adjacent residues in staphylococcal enterotoxins A and E determine T cell receptor Vβ specificity. *J. Exp. Med.* **177:** 175.

Irwin, M.J., K.R. Hudson, J.D. Fraser, and N.R.J. Gascoigne. 1992. Enterotoxin residues determining T-cell receptor Vβ binding specificity. *Nature* **359:** 841.

Janeway, C.A., J. Chalupny, P.J. Conrad, and S. Buxser. 1988. An external stimulus that mimics Mls locus responses. *J. Immunogenet.* **15:** 161.

Janeway, C.J., J. Yagi, P.J. Conrad, M.E. Katz, B. Jones, S. Vroegop, and S. Buxser. 1989. T-cell responses to Mls and to bacterial proteins that mimic its behavior. *Immunol. Rev.* **107:** 61.

Jores, R., P.M. Alzari, and T. Meo. 1990. Resolution of hypervariable regions in T-cell receptor β-chains by modified Wu-Kabat index of amino acid diversity. *Proc. Natl. Acad. Sci.* **87:** 9138.

Kappler, J.W., A. Herman, J. Clements, and P. Marrack. 1992. Mutations defining functional regions of the superantigen staphylococcal enterotoxin B. *J. Exp. Med.* **175:** 387.

Karp, D.R. and E.O. Long. 1992. Identification of HLA-DR1 beta chain residues critical for binding staphylococcal enterotoxins A and E. *J. Exp. Med.* **175:** 415.

Karp, D.R., C.L. Teletski, P. Scholl, R. Geha, and E.O. Long. 1990. The alpha 1 domain of the HLA-DR molecule is essential for high-affinity binding of the toxic shock syndrome toxin-1. *Nature* **346:** 474.

Madden, D.R., J.C. Gorga, J.L. Strominger, and D.C. Wiley. 1991. The structure of HLA-B27 reveals nonamer self-peptides bound in an extended conformation. *Nature* **353:** 321.

Marrack, P. and J. Kappler. 1990. The staphylococcal enterotoxins and their relatives. *Science* **248:** 7051.

Mollick, J.A., R.G. Cook, and R.R. Rich. 1989. Class II MHC molecules are specific receptors for staphylococcus enterotoxin A. *Science* **244:** 817.

Panina-Bordignon, P., X.T. Fu, A. Lanzavecchia, and R.W. Karr. 1992. Identification of HLA-DR α chain residues critical for binding of the toxic shock syndrome toxin superantigen. *J. Exp. Med..* **176:** 1779.

Peavy, D.L., W.H. Adler, and R.T. Smith. 1970. The mitogenic effects of endotoxin and staphylococcal enterotoxin B on mouse spleen cells and human peripheral lymphocytes. *J. Immunol.* **105:** 1453.

Pontzer, C.H., J.K. Russell, and H.M. Johnson. 1989. Localization of an immune functional site on staphylococcal enterotoxin A using the synthetic peptide approach. *J. Immunol.* **143:** 280.

———. 1991. Structural basis for differential binding of staphylococcal enterotoxin A and toxic shock syndrome toxin 1 to class II major histocompatibility molecules. *Proc. Natl. Acad. Sci.* **88:** 125.

Pontzer, C.H., M.J. Irwin, N.R.J. Gascoigne, and H.M. Johnson. 1992. T-cell antigen receptor binding sites for the microbial superantigen staphylococcal enterotoxin A. *Proc. Natl. Acad. Sci.* **89:** 7727

Purdie, K., K.R. Hudson, and J.D. Fraser. 1991. Bacterial superantigens. In *Antigen processing and presentation* (ed. J. MacCluskey), p. 193. CRC press, Boca Raton, Florida.

Russell, J.K., C.H. Pontzer, and H.M. Johnson. 1990. The I-A beta b region (65-85) is a binding site for the superantigen, staphylococcal enterotoxin A. *Biochem. Biophys. Res. Commun.* **168:** 696.

———. 1991. Both alpha-helices along the major histocompatibility complex binding cleft are required for staphylococcal enterotoxin A function. *Proc. Natl. Acad. Sci.* **88:** 7228.

Scholl, P.R., A. Diez, and R.S. Geha. 1989a. Staphylococcal enterotoxin B and toxic shock syndrome toxin-1 bind to distinct sites on HLA-DR and HLA-DQ molecules. *J. Immunol.* **143:** 2583.

Scholl, P., A. Diez, W. Mourad, J. Parsonnet, R.S. Geha, and T. Chatila. 1989b. Toxic shock syndrome toxin 1 binds to major histocompatibility complex class II molecules (published erratum appears in *Proc. Natl. Acad. Sci.* 1989 **86:** 7138). *Proc. Natl. Acad. Sci.* **86:** 4210.

Smith, D.B. and K.S. Johnson. 1988. Single step purification of polypeptides expressed in *Escherichia coli* as fusions with glutathione S-transferase. *Gene* **67:** 31.

Swaminathan, S., W. Furey, J. Pletcher, and M. Sax. 1992. Crystal structure of staphylococcal enterotoxin-B, a superantigen. *Nature* **359:** 801.

Vallee, B.L. and D.S. Auld. 1990. Active-site zinc ligands and activated H_2O of zinc enzymes. *Proc. Natl. Acad. Sci.* **87:** 220.

White, J., A. Herman, A.M. Pullen, R. Kubo, J.W. Kappler, and P. Marrack. 1989. The V beta-specific superantigen staphylococcal enterotoxin B: Stimulation of mature T cells and clonal deletion in neonatal mice. *Cell* **56:** 27.

Superantigens Expressed by Mouse Mammary Tumor Virus

H. Acha-Orbea

Ludwig Institute for Cancer Research, Lausanne Branch, 1066 Epalinges
Switzerland

ENDOGENOUS MOUSE SUPERANTIGENS

The term superantigen has been given to antigens that can interact with a large percentage of T cells. In classical antigen recognition, a complex between a processed peptide and major histocompatibility complex (MHC) molecules is recognized by the combination of all the diverse parts (Vα, Vβ, Dβ, Jα, Jβ, N-regions) of the T-cell receptor (TCR). Contrary to this, superantigens require only expression of specific TCR Vβ elements for interaction (Kappler et al. 1987a,b, 1988; Abe et al. 1988; Fry and Matis 1988; MacDonald et al. 1988; White et al. 1989). In the mouse there are about 25 Vβ elements, which explains why 1–25% of mature T cells are able to interact with a superantigen (for review, see Abe and Hodes 1989). This frequency is estimated to be about 10^4 times higher than the frequency of T cells recognizing a classical antigen. T cells interacting with a particular superantigen have a wide range of fine specificities for many different MHC peptide complexes.

Such superantigens have been found in several different pathogenic microorganisms. They include bacteria (*Staphylococci, Mycoplasma, Streptococci, Yersinia*) (Fleischer and Schrezenmeier 1988; Janeway et al. 1989; White et al. 1989; Herman et al. 1991; Stuart and Woodward 1992; for review, see Marrack and Kappler 1990), retroviruses (mouse mammary tumor virus [MMTV] [Woodland et al. 1990; 1991a,b; Acha-Orbea et al. 1991; Choi et al. 1991; Dyson et al. 1991; Frankel et al. 1991; Marrack et al. 1991; Beutner et al. 1992; Held et al. 1992; Pullen et al. 1992]), possibly murine leuke-

mia virus (Hügin et al. 1991), and possibly human immunodeficiency virus (HIV) (Imberti et al. 1992; Laurence et al.
1992), and viruses (rabies virus) (Lafon et al. 1992).

With the help of superantigens, several key steps in the development of immune tolerance have been defined. Encounter
with superantigens early in life leads to elimination of "self-
reactive" T cells in the thymus by a mechanism called clonal
deletion (Kappler et al. 1987a, 1988; MacDonald 1988). Presence of superantigens from birth leads to a hole in the T-cell
repertoire by elimination of 90–99% of the mature T cells expressing the superantigen-reactive TCR Vβ element(s). If the
first encounter happens later in life, the superantigen-reactive
T cells are activated and may initially increase in numbers (for
review, see Abe and Hodes 1989; Webb et al. 1990; Held et al.
1992). Shortly after this initial interaction, however, the
superantigen-reactive T cells are rendered unresponsive (anergic) (Rammensee et al. 1989; Webb et al. 1990). Anergic cells
are not capable of producing IL-2 in a secondary immune response. If the superantigen is continuously present after induction of anergy, peripheral as well as thymic deletion of the
superantigen-responsive T cells occurs. This results in a near-
complete loss of these T cells (Webb et al. 1990; Held et al.
1992).

In mice, many different endogenous superantigens have
been described. These endogenous superantigens (minor lymphocyte stimulating [Mls] antigens) are dominant genes found
in many different chromosomal localizations with always a
stimulating allele and a null allele (for review, see Abe and
Hodes 1989). It has recently been discovered that they are encoded by an open reading frame (*orf*) which is found in the 3'
long terminal repeat (LTR) of mouse mammary tumor virus
(MMTV) (Acha-Orbea et al. 1991a; Choi et al. 1991).

ENDOGENOUS SUPERANTIGENS ARE ENCODED BY MMTV ORF

Genetic mapping of endogenous mouse superantigens revealed
a striking linkage to endogenous proviruses of the MMTV family (Woodland et al. 1990, 1991b; Acha-Orbea et al. 1991;
Dyson et al. 1991; Frankel et al. 1991). Direct proof that
MMTV encodes these superantigens came from (1) analysis of

the TCR repertoire of transgenic mice expressing whole MMTV genomes or MMTV *orf* (Acha-Orbea et al. 1991) and (2) transfection experiments with MMTV genomes or *orf* genes (Choi et al. 1991). On the basis of these findings, it became clear that MMTV *orfs* are responsible for Mls phenotypes. Sequence alignments of translated *orf* DNA sequences revealed a striking correlation between the highly polymorphic carboxy-terminal 30 amino acids and their TCR Vβ specificity (Acha-Orbea and Palmer 1991). Overall, pORF molecules have 90–95% amino acid sequence homology.

MMTV

MMTV is a B-type retrovirus that is maternally transmitted from mother to offspring via milk. A functional immune system seems to be necessary for completion of the viral life cycle (Tsubura et al. 1988). MMTV is a major causative agent for mammary tumor development in mice (Bentvelzen and Hilgers 1980; Bentvelzen et al. 1980; Salmons and Günzberg 1987). Tumors are induced by integration close to host proto-oncogenes, which leads to their activation through the 3' LTR (Peters et al. 1983, 1986). In laboratory as well as wild mice, endogenous forms of MMTV can be found which arose by integration of MMTV into the germ line (Kozak et al. 1987). These endogenous MMTVs are inherited like normal mouse genes following Mendelian inheritance rules. The different integrated MMTV loci are called *Mtv-1*, *-2*, etc. Most of these proviruses (with the exception of *Mtv-1* to *-4*) have lost the ability to produce infectious viral particles but have retained the capacity to produce functional MMTV proteins. The different infectious and endogenous viruses show about 90–95% amino acid sequence homology. A striking feature of this retrovirus is a large LTR that contains an *orf* of about 960 base pairs overlapping with the 3' end of the envelope sequence. Besides its role as a superantigen, functions in gene regulation have been suggested (van Klaveren and Bentvelzen 1988; Salmons et al. 1990).

Although the *orf* gene product has never been demonstrated convincingly in normal lymphocytes or mammary tumor cells, the nucleotide sequence allows predictions of possible structures. As described above, the 30 carboxy-terminal amino acids seem to predict TCR Vβ specificity of the superantigen. Five in-frame start codons (ATG) are found in the amino-terminal half of the molecule. In the amino-terminal part, a hydrophobic sequence is encoded which could serve as a transmembrane (if the first ATG is used) or signal sequence (if the second ATG is used). There are five potential N-linked glycosylation sites in the amino-terminal half of the protein. In vitro translation results showed the potential of producing a type II membrane protein (Choi et al. 1992; Knight et al. 1992; Korman et al. 1992; for review, see Acha-Orbea et al. 1993).

*orf*s in a comparable localization can be found in monkey herpesvirus and HIV (*nef*). Both *nef* and *orf* have been implicated in gene regulation.

INFECTIOUS MMTVs

Parallel to the finding that endogenous MMTVs express the long-sought endogenous superantigens, it became clear that infectious viruses express superantigens as well (Acha-Orbea et al. 1991; Choi et al. 1991; Marrack et al. 1991; Held et al. 1992). Among the superantigens expressed by infectious viruses, only two (MMTV[C3H] and MMTV[GR]) affecting T cells expressing TCR Vβ14 were available at the starting point of our experiments. Both viruses were used extensively in studies on cancer until the early 1980s.

The last two years have revealed that in laboratory mice many different endogenous superantigens affecting nearly every TCR Vβ element known (with a few exceptions) could be found. When we started using MMTV(C3H) to analyze the superantigen-induced immune response in vivo, we were surprised to see only a marginal effect on Vβ14-expressing T cells in the draining lymph nodes after local injection. Although the lymph node size increased drastically shortly after injection, we observed only a weak but reproducible increase from 10% to 12% of the CD4+ T cells (Held et al. 1992).

When we did these experiments, however, we observed that about half of our commercially available BALB/c mice had strongly reduced levels of TCR Vβ6, -7, -8.1, and possibly -9. We were interested in this effect since an endogenous superantigen called Mls-1ᵃ (*Mtv-7 orf*) has the same TCR Vβ specificities and represents the strongest endogenous superantigen known. This is reflected in its capacity to induce a vigorous stimulation of the superantigen-reactive T cells in vitro and in vivo, its fast clonal deletion kinetics, and its capacity to use I-A as well as I-E molecules as presenting molecules. We characterized the new infectious MMTV(SW) in the milk of Vβ6-deleting BALB/c mice and showed that it contains an *orf* highly homologous to *Mtv-7 orf*. Strikingly, the carboxy-terminal 30 amino acids are nearly identical but very different from all the known *orfs* (Held et al. 1992), in agreement with the above stated findings.

MMTV(SW) behaves very similarly to *Mtv-7* congenic B cells when injected into naive BALB/c mice. Since BALB/c mice lack expression of a superantigen interacting with Vβ6, -7, -8.1, and -9, they express a normal repertoire of *Mtv-7* or MMTV(SW)-reactive T cells. Local injection of either leads to a fast increase in the size of draining lymph nodes. The percentage of Vβ6⁺ (superantigen-responsive) T cells increases about threefold within 4 days of injection. A single injection into naive BALB/c mice leads to a lifelong infection (Held et al. 1992). Female mice will transmit the virus to their offspring via milk, and all the injected mice will delete most of their superantigen-reactive T cells (see Table 1).

Parallel to the increase in superantigen-reactive T cells, a strong increase in the numbers of B cells is detected in the

TABLE 1 *LOCAL IMMUNE RESPONSE AFTER SUPERANTIGEN ENCOUNTER*

	Percent Vβ among CD4⁺ T cells		
	Vβ6	Vβ8.2	Vβ14
No injection	11.6	12.6	10.3
MMTV-free milk	10.7	12.9	10.4
MMTV(SW) milk	**29.6**	7.5	7.2
MMTV(C3H) milk	9.3	11.4	**12.6**
Mtv-7 B cells	**38.0**	7.7	8.4

Milk containing 4 x 10⁹ to 4 x 10¹⁰ MMTV particles or 6 x 10⁶ splenic B cells were injected into the footpads of BALB/c mice. After 4 days the draining lymph nodes were removed and analyzed by flow microfluorometry. Values showing increases of superantigen-reactive T cells are in bold type. (Reproduced from Held et al. 1992, copyright permission of the Rockefeller University Press.)

draining lymph nodes (Fig. 1). When analyzed for immunoglobulin secretion, these B cells are found to secrete large amounts of IgG. At this stage they do not require the presence of superantigen-reactive T cells for secretion of IgG anymore. Such an IgG response, however, does not take place when MMTV(SW) is injected into mice lacking superantigen-reactive T cells. Reconstitution of nude mice that lack mature T cells with superantigen-reactive T cells leads to the above-described MMTV-induced activation of B and T cells.

Analysis of the antibody isotypes secreted by these superantigen-induced B cells shows a striking predominance of IgG_{2a}, reaching peak levels around day 6 after injection (Fig. 2). For the time being, we have no direct evidence for induction of an isotype switch and terminal differentiation or for whether MMTV(SW) preferentially infects preactivated B cells expressing IgG_{2a}. This response remains localized in the draining lymph node, which starts decreasing in size around day 10 after initiation of the immune response. Thereafter, a continuous infection of the lymphocyte compartment is observed which leads to a lifelong near-complete deletion of the superantigen-responsive T cells. This IgG_{2a} response was oligo- to polyclonal (Held et al. 1993).

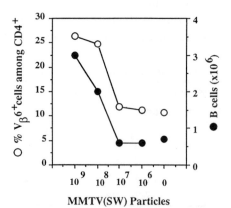

MMTV(SW) Particles

FIGURE 1 Increase of B cells and superantigen-reactive T cells after MMTV(SW)-injection. MMTV(SW) dose response curves for the increases of B (filled circles) and T cells (open circles) after local MMTV(SW) injection. The experiments were analyzed 4 days after injection. (Reprinted, with permission from Held et al. 1993, copyright permission of the Rockefeller University Press.)

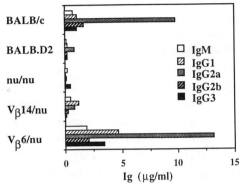

FIGURE 2 Immunoglobulin isotype secretion patterns after local MMTV(SW) injection. The draining lymph nodes of MMTV(SW)-infected BALB/c, BALB.D2 (*Mtv-7*-congenic BALB/c), BALB/c nu/nu, and BALB/c nu/nu mice reconstituted with Vβ14+ or Vβ6+ CD4+ T cells were cultured for 3 days, and the immunoglobulin-secretion patterns were determined in isotype-specific sandwich ELISAs. (Reprinted, with permission, from Held et al. 1993, copyright permission of the Rockefeller University Press.)

A striking finding of these studies was that only B cells are infected in the early phase of MMTV(SW) infection. Practically no infection can be detected in T cells (Held et al. 1993). In adult mice, however, both B and T cells have integrated copies of MMTV(SW).

MMTV(C3H) showed a very similar stimulation in the B cell but, as shown above, not in the T-cell compartment. Titration experiments indicated that this is unlikely due to lower virus titer of MMTV(C3H) as compared to MMTV(SW). We think that the I-E-dependent superantigen of MMTV(C3H) is weaker than the superantigen of MMTV(SW).

In an attempt to find other MMTVs, we screened milk of mice susceptible to mammary tumor development. So far we have been able to characterize four new MMTVs affecting T cells expressing several new TCR Vβ elements.

ANTI-ORF MONOCLONAL ANTIBODIES

When we compared the carboxy-terminal amino acid sequence of pORF of *Mtv-7* (and MMTV[SW]) with the amino acid sequence database, we found a significant degree of homology with proteins of the S-100 family. These proteins have a helix-loop-helix motif that is homologous to these carboxy-terminal *orf* sequences throughout the first helix and the loop where *orf* stops (Held et al. 1992). Since the carboxy-terminal amino acid sequence correlates so well with the TCR Vβ specificity and since such an antibody would be highly specific for both *Mtv-7* and MMTV(SW) pORF, we generated monoclonal antibodies against a peptide containing the 19 carboxy-terminal amino acid residues of pORF of *Mtv-7*. We selected five hybridomas secreting anti-pORF monoclonal antibodies as determined by ELISA using the pORF peptide. All these antibodies were able to block an in vitro Mls response completely. In addition, we demonstrated a strong reduction of clonal deletion of Mls-1[a]-reactive T cells in *Mtv-7*-expressing (Mls-1[a]) mice and a strong inhibition of the above-described lymph node response after local infection with MMTV(SW) in vivo (Fig. 3).

Using F(ab)$_2$ fragments, we failed to detect surface expression of pORF on B-cell blasts, the best Mls-presenting cells, and could not detect any pORF immunoprecipitation products. This is in contrast to recent studies of Winslow and collaborators, who used monoclonal uncleaved hamster anti-ORF peptide antibodies (Winslow et al. 1992). Our antibodies stained insect cells overexpressing the ORF protein and showed the expected precipitation products. We therefore think that very low levels of the superantigen are expressed in B-cell blasts. The results, however, clearly show that the pORF carboxy-terminal sequence is accessible on the B-cell surface (Acha-Orbea et al. 1992).

LIFE CYCLE OF VIRUS

Using the older results from the literature combined with the results of the above-described experiments, we can now begin to draw a tentative picture of the life cycle of MMTV. With a better understanding of the life cycle, we can design experiments aimed at a better understanding of the immune response.

The virus is produced in large quantities in the milk of infected mothers and enters into contact with the immune sys-

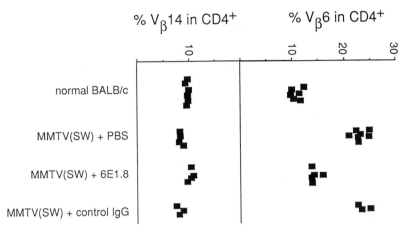

FIGURE 3 Inhibition of the anti-MMTV(SW) response by monoclonal anti-pORF antibodies in vivo. Adult BALB/c mice were injected locally with 10^7 purified MMTV(SW) particles. After 12 hr and twice a day thereafter, the mice received 50 µg of antibody in the same local site. After 4 days, the local lymph nodes were removed and analyzed by flow microfluorometry. (Reprinted, with permission, from Acha-Orbea et al. 1992, copyright permission of the Rockefeller University Press.)

tem of the newborn through the epithelial cells overlying the Peyer's patches through the gut (O. Karapetian et al., unpubl.). There the infection of lymphocytes occurs, which represents a key step for the survival of the virus. From the studies in adult mice, we suggest that the B cells are the first targets of infection and present the superantigen to T cells, and that this interaction leads to a strong amplification of the (inefficient) infection and to integration of the virus. Without this interaction the virus cannot reach sufficient levels for a continuous infection that finally results in passage to the mammary gland. Several days after infection (most likely when the immune response starts declining), the lymphocytes leave the Peyer's patches and allow the virus to enter into contact with the peripheral immune system. Infection around the time of birth may lead to a strong tolerance induction toward MMTV. At this stage, the integrated virus is hidden in infected lymphocytes. Since we can find the virus at later stages also in T cells, it must be able to jump between lymphocyte subsets. This occurs in the absence of a detectable viremia. Once the mammary gland becomes receptive for infection, the virus is capable of infecting the mammary gland. Lymphocytes are most likely the intermediate hosts for MMTV until the mammary gland becomes receptive for infection. Then the MMTV life cycle is completed. Integration (by chance) close to proto-oncogenes can lead to mammary tumor development late in life. Therefore, pORF expression fulfills the function of increasing the levels of infection with MMTV.

CONCLUDING REMARKS

Since it was discovered that MMTVs encode superantigens, it became possible to use immunological methods for a better understanding of the retrovirology and the virological methods for a better understanding of the immunology. The interplay between the two can now be used to design very sensitive and highly informative experiments in vivo. We are only at the beginning of an exciting era.

ACKNOWLEDGMENTS

I thank Werner Held, H. Robson MacDonald, Gary A. Waanders, Alexander N. Shakhov, Jean-Pierre Kraehenbuhl, and Oshine Karapetian for the many discussions and collaborations. This work was supported by a grant and a START fellowship from the Swiss National Science Foundation.

REFERENCES

Abe, R. and R. Hodes. 1989. T cell recognition of minor lymphocyte stimulating (Mls) gene products. *Annu. Rev. Immunol.* **7:** 683.

Abe, R., M.S. Vacchio, B. Fox, and R. Hodes. 1988. Preferential expression of the T-cell receptor $V_\beta 3$ gene by Mls^c reactive T cells. *Nature* **335:** 827.

Acha-Orbea, H. and E. Palmer. 1991. Mls—A retrovirus exploits the immune system. *Immunol. Today* **12:** 356.

Acha-Orbea, H., L. Scarpellino, A.N. Shakhov, W. Held, and H.R. MacDonald. 1992. Inhibition of mouse mammary tumor virus-induced T cell responses *in vivo* by antibodies to orf protein. *J. Exp. Med.* **176:** 1769.

Acha-Orbea, H., Held, W., Waanders, G.A., Shakhov, A.N., L. Scarpellino, R. Lees, and H.R. MacDonald. 1993. Exogenous and endogenous mouse mammary tumor virus superantigens. *Immunol. Rev.* **131:** 5.

Acha-Orbea, H., A.N. Shakhov, L. Scarpellino, E. Kolb, V. Müller, A. Vessaz-Shaw, R. Fuchs, K. Blöchlinger, P. Rollini, J. Billote, M. Sarafidou, H.R. MacDonald, and H. Diggelmann. 1991. Clonal deletion of $V_\beta 14$ positive T cells in mammary tumor virus transgenic mice. *Nature* **350:** 207.

Bentvelzen, P. and J. Hilgers. 1980. Murine mammary tumor virus. In *Viral oncology* (ed. G. Klein), p.311. Raven Press, New York.

Bentvelzen, P., J. Brinkhof, and F. Westenbrink. 1980. Expression of endogenous mammary tumor virus in mice: Its genetic control and relevance to spontaneous carcinogenesis. *Cold Spring Harbor Conf. Cell Proliferation* **7:** 1095.

Beutner, U., W.N. Frankel, M.S. Cote, J.M. Coffin, and B.T. Huber. 1992. Mls-1 is encoded by the long terminal repeat open reading frame of the mouse mammary tumor virus *Mtv-7*. *Proc. Natl. Acad. Sci.* **89:** 5432.

Choi, Y., J.W. Kappler, and P. Marrack. 1991. A superantigen encoded in the open reading frame of the 3' long terminal repeat of mouse mammary tumor virus. *Nature* **350:** 203.

Choi, Y., P. Marrack, and J. Kappler. 1992. Structural analysis of a mouse mammary tumor virus superantigen. *J. Exp. Med.* **175:** 847.

Dyson, P.J., A.M. Knight, S. Fairchild, E. Simpson, and K. Tomonari. 1991. Genes encoding ligands for deletion of Vβ11 T cells cosegregate with mammary tumor virus genomes. *Nature* **349:** 531.

Fleischer, B. and H. Schrezenmeier. 1988. T cell stimulation by staphylococcal enterotoxins. Clonally variable response and requirements for major histocompatibility complex class II molecules on accessory or target cells. *J. Exp. Med.* **167:** 1697.

Frankel, W.N., C. Rudy, J.M. Coffin, and B.T. Huber. 1991. Linkage of *Mls* genes to endogenous mammary tumor viruses of inbred mice. *Nature* **349:** 526.

Fry, A. M. and L.A. Matis. 1988. Self-tolerance alters T-cell receptor expression in an antigen-specific MHC-restricted immune response. *Nature* **335:** 830.

Held, W., A.N. Shakhov, S. Izui, G.A. Waanders, L. Scarpellino, H.R. MacDonald, and H. Acha-Orbea. 1993. Superantigen-reactive CD4[+] T cells are required to stimulate B cells after infection with mouse mammary tumor virus. *J. Exp. Med.* **177:**359.

Held, W., A.N. Shakhov, G. Waanders, L. Scarpellino, R. Luethy, J.-P. Kraehenbuhl, H.R. MacDonald, and H. Acha-Orbea. 1992. An exogenous mouse mammary tumor virus with properties of Mls-1[a] (*Mtv-7*). *J. Exp. Med.* **175:** 1623.

Herman, A., J.W. Kappler, P. Marrack, and A.M. Pullen. 1991. Super-antigens: Mechanism of T-cell stimulation and role in immune responses. *Annu. Rev. Immunol.* **9:** 745.

Hügin, A.W., M.S. Vacchio, and H.C. Morse III. 1991. A virus-encoded "superantigen" in a retrovirus-induced immunodeficiency syndrome in mice. *Science* **252:** 424.

Imberti, L., A. Sottini, A. Bettinardi, M. Puoti, and D. Primi. 1992. Selective depletion in HIV infection of T cells that bear specific T cell receptor Vβ sequences. *Science* **254:** 860.

Janeway, C.A., Jr., J. Yagi, P.J. Conrad, M.E. Katz, B. Jones, S. Vroegop, and S. Buxser. 1989. T-cell responses to Mls and to bacterial proteins that mimic its behavior. *Immunol. Rev.* **107:** 61.

Kappler, J.W., N. Roehm, and P. Marrack. 1987a. T cell tolerance by clonal elimination in the thymus. *Cell* **49:** 273.

Kappler, J.W., U.D. Staerz, J. White, and P.C. Marrack. 1988. Self-tolerance eliminates T cells specific for Mls-modified products of the major histocompatibility complex. *Nature* **332:** 35.

Kappler, J.W., T. Wade, J. White, W. Kushnir, M. Blackman, J. Bill, N. Roehm, and P. Marrack. 1987b. A T cell receptor V_β segment that imparts reactivity to a class II major histocompatibility complex product. *Cell* **49:** 263.

Knight, A.M., G.M. Harrison, R.J. Pease, P.J. Robinson, and P.J. Dyson. 1992. *Eur. J. Immunol.* **22:** 879.

Korman, A.J., P. Bourgarel, T. Meo, and G.E. Rieckhof. 1992. The mouse mammary tumor virus long terminal repeat encodes a type II transmembrane glycoprotein. *EMBO J.* **11:** 1901.

Kozak, C., G. Peters, R. Pauley, V. Morris, R. Michaelides, J. Dudley, M. Green, M. Davisson, O. Prakash, A. Vaidya, J. Hilgers, A. Verstraeten, N. Hynes, H. Diggelmann, D. Peterson, J.C. Cohen, C. Dickson, N. Sarkar, R. Nusse, and H. Varmus. 1987. A standardized nomenclature for endogenous mouse mammary tumor viruses. *J. Virol.* **61:** 1651.

Lafon, M., M. Lafage, A. Martinez-Arends, R. Ramirez, F. Vuiller, D. Charron, V. Lotteau, and D. Scott-Algara. 1992. Evidence for a viral superantigen in humans. *Nature* **358:** 507.

Laurence, J., A.S. Hodtsev, and D.N. Posnett. 1992. Superantigen implicated in dependence of HIV-1 replication in T cells on TCR V_β expression. *Nature* **358:** 255.

MacDonald, H.R., R. Schneider, R.L. Lees, R.K. Howe, H. Acha-Orbea, H. Festenstein, R.M. Zinkernagel, and H. Hengartner. 1988. T-cell receptor Vβ use predicts reactivity and tolerance to Mls^a-encoded antigens. *Nature* **332:** 40.

Marrack, P. and J. Kappler. 1990. The staphylococcal enterotoxins and their relatives. *Science* **248:** 705.

Marrack, P., E. Kushnir, and J. Kappler. 1991. A maternally inherited superantigen encoded by a mammary tumor virus. *Nature* **349:** 524.

Peters, G., A.E. Lee, and C. Dickson. 1986. Concerted activation of potential proto-oncogenes in carcinomas induced by mouse mammary tumor virus. *Nature* **320:** 628.

Peters, G., S. Brookes, R. Smith, and C. Dickson. 1983. Tumorigenesis by mouse mammary tumor virus: Evidence for a common region for provirus integration in mammary tumors. *Cell* **33:** 369.

Pullen, A.M., Y. Chaoi, E. Kushnir, J. Kappler, and P. Marrack. 1992. The open reading frames in the 3′ long terminal repeats of several mouse mammary tumor virus integrants encode $V_\beta 3$-specific superantigens. *J. Exp. Med.* **175:** 41.

Rammensee, H.-G., R. Kroschewsky, and B. Frangoulis. 1989. Clonal anergy induced in mature $V_\beta 6$ T lymphocytes on immunizing Mls-1^b mice with Mls-1^a expressing cells. *Nature* **339:** 541.

Salmons, B. and W.H. Günzburg. 1987. Current perspectives in the biology of mouse mammary tumor virus. *Virus Res.* **8:** 81.

Salmons, B., V. Erfle, G. Brem, and W.H. Günzburg. 1990. *naf*, a *trans*-regulating negative-acting factor encoded within the mouse mammary tumor virus open reading frame region. *J. Virol.* **64:** 6355.

Stuart, P.M. and J.G. Woodward. 1992. *Yersinia enterolytica* produces superantigen activity. *J. Immunol.* **148:** 225.

Tsubura, A., M. Inaba, S. Imai, A. Murakami, N. Oyaizu, R. Yasumizu, Y. Ohnishi, H. Tanaka, S. Morii, and S. Ikehara. 1988. Intervention of T-cells in transportation of mouse mammary tumor virus (milk factor) to mammary gland cells in vivo. *Cancer Res.* **48:** 6555.

van Klaveren, P. and P. Bentvelzen. 1988. Transactivating potential of the 3′ open reading frame of murine mammary tumor virus. *J. Virol.* **62:** 4410.

Webb, S., C. Morris, and J. Sprent. 1990. Extrathymic tolerance of mature T cells: Clonal elimination as a consequence of immunity. *Cell* **63:** 1249.

White, J., A. Herman, A.M. Pullen, R. Kubo, J.W. Kappler, and P. Marrack. 1989. The V_β-specific superantigen staphylococcal enterotoxin B: Stimulation of mature T cells and clonal deletion in neonatal mice. *Cell* **56:**27.

Winslow G., M.T. Scherer, J.W. Kappler, and P. Marrack. 1992. Detection and characterization of the mouse mammary tumor virus 7 superantigen (Mls-1a). *Cell* **71:** 719.

Woodland, D., M.P. Happ, J. Bill, and E. Palmer. 1990. Requirement for cotolerogenic gene products in the clonal deletion of I-E reactive T cells. *Science* **247:** 964.

Woodland, D.L., M.P. Happ, K.J. Gollub, and E. Palmer. 1991a. An endogenous retrovirus mediating deletion of $\alpha\beta$ T cells? *Nature* **349:** 529.

Woodland, D.L., F.E. Lund, M.P. Happ, M.A. Blackman, E. Palmer, and R.B. Corley. 1991b. Endogenous superantigen expression is controlled by mouse mammary tumor proviral loci. *J. Exp. Med.* **174:** 1255.

Superantigen Function in Mouse Mammary Tumor Virus-induced Tumorigenesis

S.R. Ross,[1] T.V. Golovkina,[1] and A. Chervonsky[2,3]

[1]Department of Biochemistry, University of Illinois College of Medicine, Chicago Illinois 60612

[2]Department of Pathology, University of Chicago, Chicago, Illinois 60637

Mouse mammary tumor virus (MMTV), one of the first on-cogenic viruses discovered, causes mammary adenocar-cinomas in mice (Heston et al. 1945). MMTV is an RNA-containing virus with a B-type morphology and can be trans-mitted exogenously as viral particles through milk (Nandi and McGrath 1973; Moore et al. 1979) or endogenously via the germ line as stably integrated proviral copies (Bentvelzen and Hilgers 1980). During lactation, the level of MMTV production dramatically increases (Bittner 1958), because transcription of integrated proviral DNA is enhanced by steroid hormone receptor recognition of sequences encoded in the long terminal repeats (LTR) of the virus (Yamamoto 1985). After infection of mammary gland cells, tumorigenesis results from integration of new copies of MMTV near cellular oncogenes, thereby ac-tivating their transcription (Fig. 1) (Nusse 1988). Thus, mice that are force-bred usually both have the highest incidence of mammary tumors and shed the largest number of viral parti-cles in their milk. Once the virus is acquired through ex-ogenous infection, it is propagated in subsequent generations.

The inbred strains of mice employed in mammary cancer research fall into three categories: (1) strains with high tumor incidence that have in situ activation in the mammary gland of endogenous proviruses (i.e., GR) (Mühlbock 1965); (2) strains

[3]Present address: Department of Immunobiology, Yale University, New Haven, Connecticut.

Superantigens: A Pathogen's View of the Immune System
© 1993 Cold Spring Harbor Laboratory Press 0-87969-398-3/93 $5 + .00

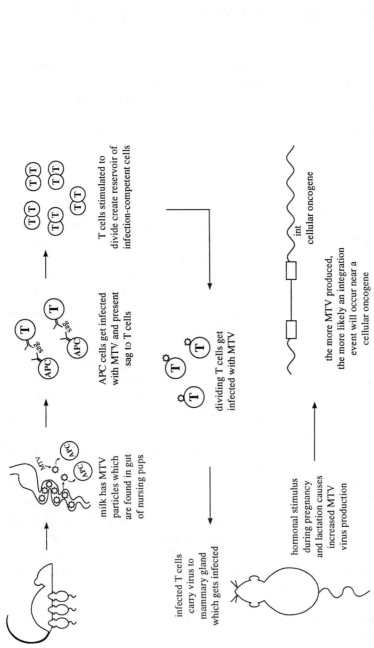

FIGURE 1 Model of acquisition of MMTV by susceptible mice leading to mammary gland tumorigenesis. (APC) Antigen-presenting cell; (sag) superantigen.

susceptible to infection by exogenous MMTV that can be freed of virus by foster-nursing on uninfected mothers (i.e., C3H/He) (Nandi and McGrath 1973); (3) resistant strains with a low incidence of mammary gland tumors in females even after nursing on viremic mothers (i.e., C57BL) (Nandi and McGrath 1973). Those strains of mice that are susceptible to exogenous MMTV-induced mammary tumors possess several characteristics in common that are associated with the immune system. For example, inbred mouse strains containing the H-2^b allele, such as C57BL, are more resistant to the exogenous virus carried by C3H/He Mtv$^+$ mice than are those with H-2^a, -2^d, -2^f, -2^k, or -2^m alleles (Mühlbock and Dux 1972). In addition, resistance to the endotoxin lipopolysaccharide (LPS) in C3H substrains has been found to be directly correlated with the level of MMTV infection and the latency of mammary tumors induced by C3H virus, with LPS-sensitive mice developing tumors at earlier times (Outzen et al. 1985).

The immune system has also been directly implicated in the infection pathway of MMTV, since neonatal thymectomy as well as splenectomy or immunosuppression can decrease or delay mammary tumor incidence (Squartini et al. 1970; Moore et al. 1979), and T (Tsubura et al. 1988) and B (Held et al. 1993) cells have both been found to carry virus. We have also found that after newborn pups nurse on viremic mothers, the thymus is the first organ in which exogenous viral RNA can be detected (T.V. Golovkina and S.R. Ross, unpubl.).

As described in detail elsewhere in this volume (Acha-Orbea; Marche et al.; Tsiagbe et al.), it has recently been discovered that MMTV proviruses encode proteins in their LTRs termed superantigens (sAg), which stimulate proliferation of specific Vβ-bearing T cells when these are recognized as foreign. Conversely, when these proviruses are inherited through the germ line, the sAg proteins cause the deletion of cognate T cells during the shaping of the immune repertoire; because of amino acid sequence variations, different MMTV loci cause the deletion of different sets of T cells in vivo. Antigen-presenting cells, such as B cells, present MMTV sAg proteins most effectively through the major histocompatibility (MHC) class II I-E molecules (Acha-Orbea and Palmer 1991).

Taken together, these data suggested to us that the MMTV

sAg protein might play a role in the ability of the virus to infect cells of the immune system. We proposed that newborn pups suckling on viremic mothers acquire exogenous MMTV, which infects cells of the immune system in the digestive tract, and that these cells carry infectious virus to the thymus (Fig. 1). Presentation of the sAg protein by either B cells or other antigen-presenting cells would therefore result in T-cell proliferation and cytokine secretion. The stimulation could create a reservoir of infection-competent cells (either the T cells themselves or bystander cells). The infected cells could then carry MMTV to the mammary gland.

The advantage of this mechanism of transmission for the virus is twofold. First, the main target tissue for MMTV infection, the epithelial cells of the mammary gland, undergo proliferation at about 4 weeks of age (during puberty) and so the virus could reside, and perhaps amplify, in cells of the immune system until this period. Second, since infection occurs during the shaping of the repertoire, those T cells bearing sAg-cognate Vβ chains are eventually deleted (Marrack et al. 1991), resulting in an immune system that could be tolerant to MMTV-infected cells at later times.

The model also predicts that endogenous MMTVs could protect mice from infection by exogenous viruses that carry the same *sag* gene by depleting cognate T cells and that these endogenous viruses might be retained as an antiviral defense mechanism. This protection would result in a decreased incidence of mammary carcinomas leading to better nursing of pups and an increased reproductive life span. Interestingly, none of the sequenced endogenous MMTV proviruses present in the genome of laboratory mice are identical to the exogenous, mammary tumor-causing MMTVs, implying that there has been a natural selection against the viruses from which the endogenous proviruses originated. Finally, the model also explains why mice containing the H-2^b allele are resistant to MMTV-induced tumors, since they lack the MHC class II I-E allele necessary for efficient viral *sag* presentation.

In this paper, we examine how expression of a *sag* transgene protects mice against MMTV-induced mammary tumors, how there is natural selection against an MMTV exogenous virus in mice that contain the same *sag* gene in their genome, and whether viral proteins other than sAg are involved in the ability of MMTV to interact with the immune system.

Does Expression of a sag Transgene Protect Mice against MMTV-induced Mammary Tumorigenesis?

We previously generated C3H/HeN inbred transgenic mice that expressed the C3H exogenous virus sAg protein under the control of the MMTV LTR (Golovkina et al. 1992) (termed MTV-ORF transgenic mice). Expression of this *sag* gene caused the deletion of Vβ14+ T cells. Transgenic females were nursed on viremic mothers and examined for evidence of viral infection, by looking for production of virus in their milk during lactation. This was accomplished by carrying out RNA histoblots (Gudkov et al. 1989) of frozen sections of their nursing pups and looking for hybridization of MMTV-specific probes to their milk-filled stomachs. Even when the transgenic mice were force-bred, we found no evidence of virus production after five pregnancies, in contrast to nontransgenic mice, which shed large amounts of virus even after the first pregnancy (Fig. 2). Thus, because the MTV-ORF transgenic mice lacked Vβ14+ T cells that were capable of being stimulated by the viral sAg protein, they could not be efficiently infected with C3H exogenous MMTV.

If endogenous MMTVs are retained in the genome of mice as an antiviral defense mechanism, the inability to be infected should result in an elimination or decrease in mammary tumor incidence. The C3H/HeN strain of mice is highly susceptible to MMTV infection and mammary tumors; in our experiments, the age at which 50% of the nontransgenic mice infected through milk developed mammary tumors was about 225 days; 90% of the females had tumors before 10 months. In contrast, MTV-ORF transgenic C3H/HeN mice that were infected with virus through nursing on the same mothers had a much longer latency and lower incidence of mammary tumors; 50% tumor incidence occurred at about 1 year, whereas at 10 months, only 25% had developed mammary tumors. The majority of the tumors in the transgenic mice were the result of new integrations of C3H exogenous virus (T. Golovkina et al., in prep.).

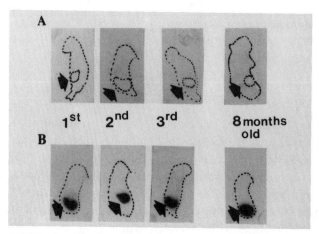

FIGURE 2 MTV-ORF transgenic mice do not produce detectable MMTV in their milk. Shown are histoblots of the newborn offspring of MMTV-infected MTV-ORF transgenic (*A*) and nontransgenic C3H/HeN Mtv+ (*B*) mice. 1st, 2nd, and 3rd denote which pregnancy the offspring came from; at the age of 8 months (5th pregnancy), the nontransgenic C3H/HeN Mtv+ female developed a mammary tumor.

Loss of Milk-borne MMTV from the MTV-ORF Transgenic Pedigree; Natural Selection in the Laboratory

Although the MTV-ORF transgenic mice did not get MMTV-induced mammary tumors at the same latency and frequency as nontransgenic mice, there was still enough virus "leaking" through to cause later development of these tumors. The development of such tumors was at late enough times not to have an impact on the reproductive life span of mice in the wild, since most feral mice do not live longer than 1 year. The presence of the endogenous *sag* gene was therefore sufficient to greatly reduce, but not completely eliminate, MMTV infection from animals.

Inheritance of the *sag* gene through multiple generations, however, resulted in complete elimination of MMTV from mice. Since viral infection in the transgenic mice was undetectable by hybridization techniques, we instead used a more sensitive method to determine whether mice were infected, by quantitating the percentage of cognate Vβ14+ T cells in their immune repertoire (Fig. 3) (exogenous virus infection results in deletion of these cells by 5 months of age [A, D, F, and I, Fig. 3]

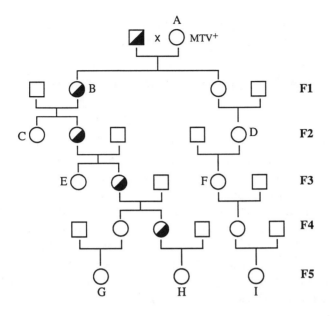

Mouse	CD4+/Vβ14+
A	1.90 ± 0.3
B	1.20 ± 0.2
C	2.00 ± 0.5
D	1.90 ± 0.05
E	4.30 ± 0.1
F	2.10 ± 0.05
G	8.75 ± 0.35
H	8.05 ± 0.05
I	2.30 ± 0.3
C3H MTV⁻	8.20 ± 0.2

FIGURE 3 Milk-borne MMTV is lost from a MTV-ORF transgenic pedigree. T cells were isolated from peripheral blood of the mice indicated and were analyzed for the percentage of CD4+/Vβ14+ cells. The numbers shown represent the average of 2–3 mice 5 months of age.

[Marrack et al. 1991; Ignatowicz et al. 1992]). At the F_2 generation, virus was transmitted from a transgenic mother to her nontransgenic offspring, which showed a high deletion of Vβ14+ cells (C in Fig. 3). By the F_3 generation, much less virus was transmitted, since the level of deletion of these T cells was 50% that seen in the F_2 mice (compare C and E in Fig. 3) and virus was completely eliminated by the F_5 generation in the transgenic mouse lineage (compare G, H, and I in Fig. 3).

The MMTV Envelope Gene May Participate in sag Stimulation of T Cells In Vivo

Deletion of cognate T cells by a transgene that contained the *sag* gene reduced and delayed the incidence of MMTV-induced mammary tumors. Nonetheless, the transgenic mice were not completely free of virus. We examined next whether there was any reservoir of cells in these animals that could be stimulated by virus. Although MTV-ORF mice lacked detectable $V\beta14^+$ peripheral T cells, in contrast to the permanent deletion of cognate thymocytes induced by endogenous MMTV proviruses, none of the *sag*-expressing transgenic adult mice showed deletion of their $V\beta14^+$ thymocytes (Table 1). Newborn MTV-ORF mice did have this deletion, however (Table 1) (Golovkina et al. 1992); the reappearance of $V\beta14^+$ T cells in the thymus glands of MTV-ORF mice began at about day 10 after birth and was complete by 2 months (T. Golovkina et al., in prep.). This indicated that the *sag* gene alone was insufficient for permanent deletion of cognate thymocytes and that its inability to completely protect against viral infection could be the result of this.

Interestingly, all of the endogenous MMTV proviruses studied to date appear to contain all four of the viral genes (*gag*, *pol*, *env*, and *sag*), with the exception of endogenous provirus *Mtv-6*, which contains two LTRs and a small region of the *env* gene (Kozak et al. 1987). This suggests that there might be some selection for the retention of viral genes in addition to *sag* in endogenous proviruses.

To test the role of the other MMTV genes in thymic deletion, a transgenic strain Hybrid Provirus (HYB PRO) was made, containing an entire copy of an MMTV provirus in which the 5' half (including the 5' LTR, *gag*, and *pol* genes) was derived from the *Mtv-1* endogenous locus present in C3H/HeN mice and the 3' half (including the 3' LTR, *env*, and *sag* genes) came from C3H exogenous virus (Shackleford and Varmus 1988). This strain contains 1–2 copies of the transgene (T. Golovkina et al., in prep.).

TABLE 1 DELETION OF Vβ14+ T CELLS IN MTV-ORF AND HYB PRO TRANSGENIC MICE

| Mice | CD4+ T cells bearing Vβ14(%)[a] | | |
	peripheral[b] (adult)	newborn	thymus[c] adult[d]
C3H/He MMTV (−)	8.2 ± 1.1	0.44 ± 0.03	0.45 ± 0.02
C3H/He MMTV (+)	3.0 ± 0.9 (37%)	0.59 ± 0.12	0.17 ± 0.03 (47%)
ORF 16H	1.2 ± 0.2 (15%)	0.09 ± 0.01 (20%)	0.45 ± 0.02
ORF 35	1.8 ± 0.4 (22%)	0.10 ± 0.02 (23%)	0.4[e]
ORF 13	2.1 ± 0.2 (26%)	not done	0.38[e]
HYB PRO	1.1 ± 0.5 (13%)	0.1[e] (23%)	0.09 ± 0.05 (20%)

[a] T cells were isolated from the peripheral blood, lymph node, or thymus of the mice indicated and analyzed for percentages of CD4-bearing Vβ14+ cells. The numbers shown represent the average of between 2 and 4 animals. Numbers in parentheses represent the percentage of Vβ14+ cells relative to the C3H/He MMTV(−) animals.
[b] The mice analyzed were 3–5 months old.
[c] Numbers shown are the Vβ14 high, CD4+ cells.
[d] The mice analyzed were 5 months old.
[e] Numbers represent the data from one animal.

Like the MTV-ORF transgenic mice, the HYB PRO transgenic mice showed specific deletion of both CD4⁺/Vβ14⁺ and CD8⁺/Vβ14⁺ T cells, and we could see this deletion in the thymuses of newborn mice (Table 1). However, the Vβ14-bearing T cells from the thymuses of adult HYB PRO transgenic mice, as well as from age-matched C3H/HeN Mtv⁺ mice, were present in significantly lower amounts than they were in the C3H/HeN Mtv⁻ nontransgenic or adult MTV-ORF mice.

These results indicated that sAg presentation to cognate thymocytes was not as effective in MTV-ORF mice as it was in the case of mice expressing endogenous MMTVs, the HYB PRO transgene, or exogenous MMTV. To investigate whether there were differences in the ability to present sAg protein among these mice, we determined whether splenocytes from these animals could stimulate the proliferation of either C3H/HeN MMTV⁻ nontransgenic primary spleen cells or Vβ14- and Vβ15-bearing T-cell hybridomas (both the Vβ14 and Vβ15 chains of the T-cell receptor interact with the C3H MMTV sAg protein [Choi et al. 1991]). The spleen cells from MTV-ORF transgenic mice could not stimulate IL-2 production by either Vβ14- or Vβ15-bearing T-cell hybridomas (Fig. 4) or proliferation of C3H/HeN MMTV⁻ nontransgenic spleen cells (T. Golovkina et al., in prep.), whereas HYB PRO spleen cells caused a considerable response of either type of responder cell (Fig. 4). The difference in the ability to respond was not due to the level of expression of the *sag* gene in HYB PRO and MTV-ORF splenocytes, because RNase T_1 protection assays using a probe specific to the MTV-ORF and HYB PRO transgenes showed that the level of *sag* RNA was higher in the MTV-ORF than HYB PRO transgenic mice (T. Golovkina et al., in prep.). Moreover, the MTV-ORF transgenic splenocytes, which are deleted for sAg-cognate T cells, did not respond to the HYB PRO splenocytes, indicating that this reaction was directed to the sAg protein (not shown). The only genetic difference between the MTV-ORF and HYB PRO transgenic mice is the presence of the exogenous C3H MMTV *env* gene, since the other two genes (*gag* and *pol*) of the HYB PRO transgene are derived from the *Mtv-1* endogenous provirus already present in the genome of C3H/HeN mice. Therefore, the *env* gene may be involved in the presentation of the sAg protein in vivo.

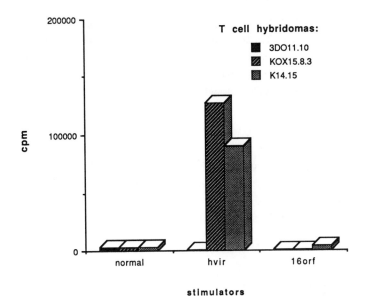

stimulators

FIGURE 4 IL-2 production by Vβ14 and Vβ15 T-cell hybridomas can be stimulated by HYB PRO but not MTV-ORF spleen cells. ^{3}H-Thymidine incorporation (cpm) by an IL-2-dependent cell line was used to measure IL-2 production. The T-cell hybridomas expressed the Vβ8.2 (3DO11.10), Vβ15 (KOX15.8.3), and Vβ14 (K14.15) T-cell receptor chains. Abbreviation: (hvir) HYBPRO; (16orf) MTV-ORF. (Choi et al. 1991).

DISCUSSION

The *sag* gene is critical to the ability of MMTV to infect mice and cause mammary tumors, most likely because its presentation to cognate T cells results in their proliferation, leading to viral infection of stimulated cells of the immune system. Conversely, mice that retain endogenous MMTV proviruses lack T cells capable of responding to certain sAg proteins and are not efficiently infected with exogenous viruses which produce sAg proteins of the same T-cell specificity. As a result, these mice are protected against early mammary tumors and do not efficiently transmit exogenous virus to their offspring. Exogenous viruses that are not efficiently transmitted are lost after several generations of passage through such mice.

Infection of cells by retroviruses occurs when the envelope protein expressed on the surface of the virus binds to a cellular receptor. In the case of MMTV, it is not known what cell-surface protein acts as the viral receptor. Our results indicate that the envelope protein may also participate in the presentation of sAg protein to T cells. What role the envelope protein plays in this presentation awaits further studies.

ACKNOWLEDGMENTS

We thank J. Prescott and P. Wright for help with some of the experiments and D. Ting for the illustrations. This work was supported by Public Health Service grant CA-45954. T.V.G is a fellow of the Cancer Research Institute.

REFERENCES

Acha-Orbea, H. and E. Palmer. 1991. Mls: A retrovirus exploits the immune system. *Immunol. Today* **12:** 356.

Bentvelzen, P. and J. Hilgers. 1980. Murine mammary tumor virus. In *Viral oncology* (ed. G. Klein), p.311. Raven Press, New York.

Bittner, J.J. 1958. Genetic concepts in mammary cancer in mice. *Ann. N.Y. Acad. Sci.* **71:** 943.

Choi, Y., J.W. Kappler, and P. Marrack. 1991. A superantigen encoded in the open reading frame of the 3′ long terminal repeat of the mouse mammary tumor virus. *Nature* **350:** 203.

Golovkina, T.V., A. Chervonsky, J.P. Dudley, and S.R. Ross. 1992. Transgenic mouse mammary tumor virus superantigen expression prevents viral infection. *Cell* **69:** 637.

Gudkov, A.V., K.N. Kashkin, T.E. Zaitsevskaya, and S. Troyanovsky. 1989. Histo-blotting: Hybridization in situ detection of specific RNAs on tissue sections transferred on nitrocellulose. *Int. J. Cancer* **44:** 1052.

Held, W., A.N. Shaknow, S. Izui, G.A. Waanders, L. Scarpellino, H.R. MacDonald, and H. Acha-Orbea. 1993. Superantigen-reactive CD4+ T cells are required to stimulate B cells after infection with mouse mammary tumor virus. *J. Exp. Med.* **177:** 359.

Heston, W.E., M.K. Deringer, and H.B. Andervont. 1945. Gene-milk agent relationship in mammary tumor development. *J. Natl. Cancer Inst.* **5:** 289.

Ignatowicz, L., J.W. Kappler, and P. Marrack. 1992. The effects of chronic infection with a superantigen-producing virus. *J. Exp. Med.* **175:** 917.

Kozak C., G. Peters, R. Pauley, V. Morris, R. Michalides, J. Dudley, M. Green, M. Davisson, O. Prakash, A. Vaidya, J. Hilgers, A. Verstraeten, N. Hynes, H. Diggelmann, D. Peterson, J.C. Cohen, C. Dickson, N. Sarkar, R. Nusse, H. Varmus, and R. Callahan. 1987. A standardized nomenclature for endogenous mouse mammary tumor viruses. *J. Virol.* **61:** 1651.

Marrack, P., E. Kushnir, and J. Kappler. 1991. A maternally inherited superantigen encoded by mammary tumor virus. *Nature* **349:** 524.

Moore, D.H., C.A. Long, A.B. Vaidya, J.B. Sheffield, A.S. Dion, and E.Y. Lasfargues. 1979. Mammary tumor viruses. *Adv. Cancer Res.* **29:** 347.

Mühlbock, O. 1965. Note on a new inbred mouse strain GR/A. *Eur. J. Cancer* **1:** 123.

Mühlbock, O. and A. Dux. 1972. MTV-variants and histocompatibility. In *Fundamental research on mammary tumours* (ed. J. Mouriquand), p.11. INSERM, Paris.

Nandi S. and C.M. McGrath. 1973. Mammary neoplasia in mice. *Adv. Cancer Res.* **17:** 353.

Nusse, R. 1988. The int genes in mammary tumorigenesis and in normal development. *Trends Genet.* **4:** 291.

Outzen, H.C., D. Corrow, and L.D. Shultz. 1985. Attenuation of exogenous murine mammary tumor virus virulence in the C3H/HeJ mouse substrain bearing the Lps mutation. *J. Natl. Cancer Inst.* **75:** 917.

Shackleford, G.M. and H.E. Varmus. 1988. Construction of a clonable, infectious, and tumorigenic mouse mammary tumor virus provirus and a derivative genetic vector. *Proc. Natl. Acad. Sci.* **85:** 9655.

Squartini, F., M. Olivi, and G.B. Bolis. 1970. Mouse strain and breeding stimulation as factors influencing the effect of thymectomy on mammary tumorigenesis. *Cancer Res.* **30:** 2069.

Tsubura, A., M. Inaba, S. Imai, A. Murakami, N. Oyaizu, R. Yasumizu, Y. Ohnishi, H. Tanaka, S. Morii, and S. Ikehara. 1988. Intervention of T-cells in transportation of mouse mammary tumor virus (milk factor) to mammary gland cells in vivo. *Cancer. Res.* **48:** 6555.

Yamamoto K.R. 1985. Steroid receptor regulated transcription of specific genes and gene networks. *Annu. Rev. Genet.* **19:** 209.

Polymorphism of TCR Vβ Regions and Clonal Deletions in Wild Mouse Populations

P.N. Marche, E. Jouvin-Marche, and P.-A. Cazenave
Unité d'Immunochimie Analytique, Département d'Immunologie
Institut Pasteur (UA CNRS 359 and Université Pierre et Marie Curie)
75724 Paris Cedex 15, France

T cells recognize antigens by a specific receptor (TCR) which is composed of two disulfide-linked polypeptide chains, α and β (Davis and Bjorkman 1988). The variable domains (V) of each chain bear the antigen specificity and are generated during T-lymphocyte ontogeny by somatic rearrangements between different gene segments. The TCR Vβ domains are encoded by Vβ, Dβ, and Jβ, but no D element has been found in the Vα domains. In the mouse, molecular cloning and statistical analyses have given an estimate that there are about 30 Vβ gene segments (Chou et al. 1987; Six et al. 1991) and 75–100 Vα segments (Arden et al. 1985; Jouvin-Marche et al. 1989). The usage of Vβ domains can be precisely determined by means of monoclonal antibodies that react specifically with Vβ regions. Using this analysis, it was shown that superantigens, such as minor lymphocyte stimulatory (Mls) and bacterial toxins, stimulate subsets of T lymphocytes that express particular Vβ regions with little or no influence from the other TCR elements (Janeway et al. 1989; White et al. 1989). The expression of endogenous superantigens leads to the dramatic depletion of reactive T cells during the development of T cells in the thymus. This results in the absence in mature T lymphocytes of T-cell subsets bearing the target Vβ domains, a phenomenon called "clonal deletion" (Kappler et al. 1988; MacDonald et al. 1988; Herman et al. 1991; Janeway 1991). Recently, it has been established that mouse mammary tumor virus (MMTV) transmitted in milk of certain C3H individuals encodes super-antigen that controls the levels of Vβ14 T cells (Marrack et al. 1991). So far, all Mls antigens and endogenous superantigens have been shown to be encoded by MMTV that was integrated in the mouse genome and then to be transmitted as Mtv loci following Mendelian rules. The coding region of the super-antigen consists of an open reading frame located in the 3′ long terminal repeat (LTR) of Mtv (Acha-Orbea et al. 1991; Choi et al. 1991; Dyson et al. 1991; Frankel et al. 1991; Mar-rack et al. 1991; Woodland et al. 1991).

Vβ usages in T cells were studied in some prototype laboratory strains of mice that are used as models for response or pathology. Such a limited set of strains cor-responds to a reduced sample of individuals; therefore, general conclusions are most probably biased. Currently, we are ex-tending the analysis of Vβ usages in a large panel of wild-derived strains and wild trapped mice with the aim of determining the variations of Vβ expression, defining factors affecting the levels of Vβ, and evaluating the significance of clonal deletion phenomena in natural populations.

WILD MICE

The mice used in our studies originated in Eurasia and belong to the *Mus musculus* species, which is one of the four species of the genus, along with *M. spretus*, *M. spicilegus*, and *M. ab-botti* (Bonhomme and Guénet 1989). *M. musculus* is a complex species that includes four main subspecies: *M. m. domesticus*, *M. m. musculus*, *M. m. bactrianus*, and *M. m. castaneus*. (A subspecies is defined as an entity showing a differentiated gene pool while retaining the ability to intercross with other such entities [Bonhomme and Guénet 1989]). *M. musculus* species originated in the Indian subcontinent, from where it has emigrated to colonize all the major geographical areas of Eurasia (W. Din et al., in prep.). A limited number of individu-als of *M. musculus* species gave rise to the laboratory strains of mice.

We are studying inbred strains derived from wild individu-als trapped in Europe that belong to *M. m. domesticus* and *M.*

m. musculus subspecies. In addition, individuals from natural populations of different geographical areas in eastern Europe and Asia were included in our studies.

DIFFERENTIAL USAGE OF Vβ DOMAINS IN MICE

Studies of the TCR β locus have revealed that the Vβ gene segments can be grouped in subfamilies based on sequence similarities. These subfamilies are composed predominantly of a single member, except for Vβ5 and Vβ8, which both have three members. As a consequence of this relatively simple organization, the Vβ gene segments display great structural divergence, thus explaining why monoclonal antibodies specific for single Vβ domains were obtained for a great number of Vβ regions. The general organization of the mouse Vβ subfamilies is depicted in Figure 1. In the laboratory BALB/c strain, which can be considered as a reference, 24 of the 29 Vβ gene segments so far described are organized in 20 subfamilies. Five Vβ segments, which were described as pseudo-

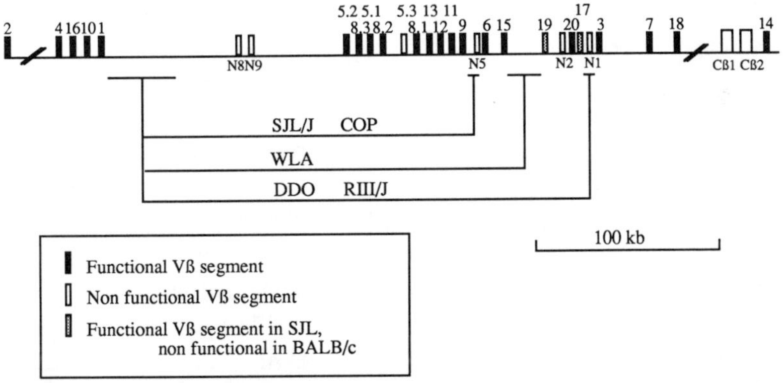

FIGURE 1 Organization of the TCR β chain locus. Each block represents a Vβ gene segment that is identified above the diagram. The two constant region genes and the five V gene segments possessing heavy alterations in their coding regions are indicated below. The extent of the germ-line deletions observed in some mice are shown by horizontal lines. The organization is derived from Malissen et al. (1986); Chou et al. (1987); Haqqi et al. (1989); Jouvin-Marche et al. (1989); Louie et al. (1989); Six et al. (1991).

gene segments, have not yet been attributed to any structural subfamily (Louie et al. 1989). The number of Vβ regions actually utilized differs greatly among the different laboratory strains of mice and is dependent on several factors. First, polymorphism of some Vβ gene segments may account for differential usage; for instance, Vβ17 and Vβ19 are pseudogenes in mice of TCRβ^b haplotype as BALB/c and are functional in mice of TCRβ^a haplotype as SJL (Wade et al. 1988; Louie et al. 1989). Second, several strains of mice display genomic deletions in the TCR β locus that remove contiguous Vβ gene segments, as in the laboratory strain SJL (Behlke et al. 1986). Several deletions were found among wild-derived strains or individuals that lack up to two-thirds of their Vβ gene segments, as in RIII/J strain (Haqqi et al. 1989) and DDO individuals (Jouvin-Marche et al. 1989). Finally, along with this variability in the content of Vβ germ-line gene segments, the usage of Vβ regions by peripheral T lymphocytes depends on MHC products and on the expression of superantigens that lead to clonal elimination of T cells bearing TCR using particular Vβ regions (Abe and Hodes 1989). The number of Vβ regions whose expression is affected by clonal deletion phenomena is still not definitive, and to date one can estimate that at least a dozen Vβ regions are targets of superantigens that act as Vβ-deleting elements (Vβ-DE).

To evaluate the consequence of the lack of Vβ gene segments, we have analyzed in the mice displaying germ-line deletions the expression of the remaining Vβ for which antibodies were available: Vβ2 (Necker et al. 1991), Vβ3 (Pullen et al. 1988), Vβ4 (Tomonari et al. 1990), Vβ6 (Kanagawa et al. 1989), Vβ7 (Okada et al. 1990), Vβ14 (Liao et al. 1989), and Vβ17 (Kappler et al. 1987). We did not include anti-Vβ10 monoclonal antibodies in our studies because they are known to react only with some Vβ10 alleles (Necker et al. 1991; Tomonari and Hengartner 1992) and thus do not recognize some Vβ10 alleles from wild, as we observed in WLA and COP strains. The mice were bled at the retro-orbital sinus, and blood was collected on heparine. Lymphocytes were isolated by Ficoll purification. Double stainings were performed as described previously (Cazenave et al. 1990; Jouvin-Marche et al. 1992b) on 1–2 million cells that were incubated with FITC-labeled monoclonal antibodies anti-CD3 (Leo et al. 1987) and with biotinylated labeled monoclonal antibodies anti-Vβ followed by R-streptavidin-phycoerythrine staining. Cytofluoranalysis was performed with a FACScan analyzer (Becton and Dickinson). In Table 1, representative results are presented. CBA/J strain has the same Vβ haplotype as BALB/c and therefore does not have germ-line deletion. The lack of Vβ3 T lymphocytes is due to a clonal deletion controlled by Mtv-3 integrated in the CBA/J genome. SJL strain expresses significantly all the Vβ tested. COP strain has the same Vβ haplotype as SJL and displays a pattern of Vβ expression quite similar to that of SJL within the range of experimental incertitude, with the exception of Vβ6, whose level of expression is reduced in COP. The WLA strain lacks two functional gene segments as compared to SJL or COP strains, is devoid of Vβ3 T cells, and expresses an increased level of Vβ4 T cells, whereas the other Vβ levels are not affected. DDO mice are not inbred, and variations in Vβ utilization are observed between different individuals, especially for Vβ2 and Vβ4. In all DDO individuals, the levels of Vβ7 and Vβ14 expression are in the same range, and as found in the WLA strain, no Vβ3 T cells were detected. It is interesting to note that in DDO mice three Vβ gene segments, namely Vβ2, Vβ4, and Vβ14, account for the majority of the peripheral T cells: up to 60%. Furthermore, if the DDO1 individual has a

TABLE 1 EXPRESSIONS OF Vβ DOMAIN DETERMINED IN PERIPHERAL BLOOD BY CYTOFLUOROMETRY

	Vβ2	Vβ3	Vβ4	Vβ6	Vβ7	Vβ14	Vβ17	I-E
CBA/J	9	0	12	0.6	0.7	10	n.d.	+
SJL	14	3.5	14	11.8	2.7	7.6	9.3	−
COP	8.8	2.4	14.8	4.6	4.4	8.4	13	−
WLA	9	0	22	GD	4	10	n.d.	+
DDO1	4.1	0	33	GD	0	13	GD	+
DDO4	26	0	21	GD	0.9	11	GD	+
DDO5	26	0	20	GD	1.4	12	GD	+

Numbers indicate the percentages of CD3 T cells bearing the indicated Vβ. + indicates the presence of the class II molecules. The expression of the Vβ17 domain was not done for CBA/J and WLA strains, indicated by n.d., because both strains have the nonfunctional Vβ17 gene segment. GD stands for germ-line deletion of the corresponding Vβ gene segment.

low percentage of Vβ2 T cells, then Vβ4 is expressed by one third of the T cells. Taken together, these data indicate that in some wild mice, the number of Vβ gene segments used to elaborate the T-cell repertoire could be reduced.

Mtv IN WILD MICE

Superantigens related to the Mls antigens are encoded by a wide variety of integrated Mtv genomes in the common laboratory strains and in mice isolated from wild populations (Pullen et al. 1988, 1990; Bill et al. 1989; Singer et al. 1990; Vacchio et al. 1990; Woodland et al. 1990; Jouvin-Marche et al. 1992b). Analysis of the laboratory strains indicated that the number of the integration copies of MMTV genomes varies greatly and that the polymorphism of the integration sites is extensive (Callahan et al. 1982; Frankel et al. 1991; Jouvin-Marche et al. 1992a). So far, about 50 different endogenous Mtv loci have been identified in the laboratory strains (Kozak et al. 1987; Tomonari et al 1993). The endogenous Mtv loci are detected by Southern blot using a probe derived from the envelope gene of the MMTV-C3H genome (Majors and Varmus 1983). The complexity of the hybridizing patterns is very variable among the wild mice and is not dependent on their geographical origin or their level of inbreeding. Some strains display a complex pattern of six to nine visible hybridizing fragments; others have very few copies of endogenous MMTV. Finally, two wild-derived inbred strains, 38CH and MOL, are free of endogenous MMTV (Jouvin-Marche et al. 1992a). Figure 2 represents hybridization patterns obtained after *Eco*RI digestion of genomic DNA from mice displaying genomic deletions in the TCR β locus. The inbred strains SJL, COP, and WLA contain one or two fragments hybridizing with the envelope probe. SJL is known to possess Mtv-8 and Mtv-51. COP contains three endogenous Mtv: Mtv-13, -14, and -17, located on chromosome 4. These integrants can be distinguished by a probe corresponding to the LTR (not shown). The Mtv of WLA is under investigation. In contrast, the DDO mice display a large number of hybridizing fragments; the individuals presented in Figure 2 are representative of the pattern of hybridization obtained.

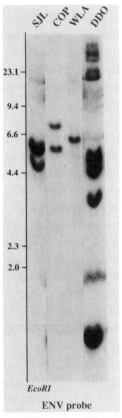

FIGURE 2 Southern blot analysis of integrated Mtv genomes. Genomic DNA (12–15 μg) was digested by *EcoRI*, and the fragments were separated in 0.7% agarose gel and then analyzed by Southern analysis using a ^{32}P-labeled MMTV envelope probe consisting of a 2.3-kb *HindIII-BglII* fragment (Majors and Varmus 1983). The sizes in kilobases of the λ *HindIII* fragments are indicated on the left.

CLONAL DELETIONS

The nondetection of T cells bearing a given Vβ region in mice possessing the corresponding functional gene segment can be due either to allelic polymorphism altering the epitope recognized by the anti-Vβ monoclonal antibodies or to a deleting element inducing the clonal deletion of T cells bearing this Vβ domain. This can be analyzed by mating the animals that express the tested Vβ region with those that do not. If offspring of such crosses do not express the Vβ domain, that demonstrates that the nonexpression phenotype is due to the inheritance of a dominant genetic character that controls the clonal elimination of the target T cells. By the analyses of F_2 crosses, it is possible to determine whether the nonexpression follows the segregation of an endogenous Mtv.

To investigate whether the low level of Vβ2 expression in some DDO individuals is due to the presence of a superantigen acting as Vβ2-DE, such genetic analyses were carried out. DDO mice having few $Vβ2^+CD3^+$ T cells were crossed with the SJL strain, which has a significant level of Vβ2 T cells. F_1 hybrids lack $Vβ2^+CD3^+$ T cells, as the DDO parent. To identify the putative Mtv integrants controlling the expression of Vβ2, the segregations of endogenous Mtv were analyzed in F_2 animals. The genetic linkage analysis was completed by crossing one F_2 individual that displays the non-expressor phenotype with an SBK mouse that has no Mtv integrants and expresses Vβ2 at a level similar to that of the SJL strain. Repeated crosses with mice devoid of endogenous Mtv led to the identification of a 5-kb *Eco*RI fragment hybridizing with the Mtv probe whose presence correlated precisely with the deletion of Vβ2 T cells. All progenies lacking this Mtv expressed significant levels of Vβ2 T cells. Taken together, the data of the Mtv segregation and the pattern of Vβ2 expression show that a Mtv integrant present in the 5-kb *Eco*RI fragment, Mtv-DDO, controls the level of Vβ2 expression, and therefore is a Vβ2-DE. Furthermore, the presence of I-E molecules does not affect Vβ2 expression, since some I-E-negative individuals have a low percentage of Vβ2 T cells. This indicates that Vβ2-DE can be efficiently presented by I-A molecules.

In the course of analysis of Vβ17 TCR expression in inbred strains derived from populations of wild mice, we found that (PWK x CBA/J) F_1 progenies and the wild-derived mouse strain MAI, which expresses I-E and possesses Vβ17a2 allele, deletes Vβ17 T cells in mature repertoires (Cazenave et al. 1990). This indicates that CBA/J and MAI have self-superantigens interacting with Vβ17a2 T cells. We followed Vβ17 expression and segregation of endogenous Mtv from CBA/J and MAI in three sets of backcross hybrids. The deletion of the Vβ17a2 T cells precisely correlates with the presence of Mtv-6 from CBA/J and a Mtv from MAI (Jouvin-Marche et al. 1992b). Mtv-6 is known to control Mls3 expression, which is associated with the strongest Vβ3 deletion (Frankel et al. 1991). In the backcrosses, Vβ3 expression follows precisely that of Vβ17, thus confirming the Mls3 phenotype, indicating that Vβ3⁺ T cells of PWK are deleted by Mtv-6 and that Mtv-MAI deletes Vβ3⁺ T cells as well. Furthermore, all the progenies displaying Mtv-6 delete Vβ17a2 T cells, irrespective of the expression of H-2 I-E. These data show that superantigens related to MMTV control Vβ17a2 expression independently of the expression of I-E.

The effects of Mtv-13, -14, and -17 of the COP strain and that of the Mtv of the WLA strain are under investigation. Mtv-13 induces a partial deletion of T cells bearing Vβ3 (Frankel et al. 1991), but in COP the level of Vβ3 expression is of the same range as that of SJL, which does not delete Vβ3 T cells (Table 1). This can be due either to polymorphism of the Vβ3 gene segment of COP or to differential efficiencies of the Mtv-13 from different strains.

INFLUENCE OF THE POLYMORPHISM OF Vβ GENES ON CLONAL DELETION

In laboratory strains of mice, two alleles of Vβ17 gene are found; the most frequent corresponds to a nonfunctional form (Vβ17^b) as in BALB/c (Fig. 1). This feature allows a rapid analysis of the expression of Vβ17 genes present in the wild mice, by crosses with the laboratory strains bearing Vβ17^b. Our study of Vβ17 polymorphism by Southern blot revealed eight different restriction fragments among about 200 tested mice that were trapped in the wild (Jouvin-Marche et al. 1992a). Populations of mice from India display large polymorphism and include the eight fragments, whereas in populations from other places, one or two fragments were found. From this sample, we have determined the structure of four allelic forms of the Vβ17 domain that were not found in laboratory strains. The substitutions among the Vβ17 alleles are all localized either in the FR3 and/or in the CDR2 loops. The impact of these variant residues on the Vβ17 specificity toward self-superantigens was studied in F_1 and F_2 hybrids with laboratory strains. Only the substitutions in FR3 affect Vβ reactivity, confirming that the interactions of TCR with superantigens or peptide/ MHC complexes involve distinct regions of the TCR. Estimation of the Vβ17 allele frequencies indicates that Vβ17a1, found in laboratory mice, is rare in wild populations, whereas the Vβ17a2 allele first described in the PWK strain (Cazenave et al. 1990) is the most frequent allele. Our data suggest that Vβ17 allele diversification is not driven by reactivity with endogenous superantigens, since most of the differences among Vβ17 alleles are in the CDR2, which is not crucial in superantigen recognition.

STRUCTURE OF THE ENDOGENOUS SUPERANTIGENS

Based on sequence comparisons of the last 30 amino acids, Mtv can be divided into structural groups that correlate generally with the specificities toward target Vβ. The structures of Vβ3-DE were determined from Mtv-1, -3, -6, -13, and -MAI (Fig. 3). Mtv-1, -6, and -13 are identical, and Mtv-6 displays a single amino acid difference. Mtv-MAI, acting as Vβ17a2 and Vβ3-DE, is significantly more divergent in the first half of the carboxy-terminal region, whereas the second half is highly conserved. Indeed, a stretch of 11 residues is conserved among all these Mtv (Jouvin-Marche et al. 1992b). Further studies of the structure of Mtv-DDO, which deletes Vβ2, confirm this observation (E. Jouvin-Marche et al., in prep.). In this region, Mtv-DDO displays two amino acid changes that may be responsible for the shift of the Vβ specificity (Fig. 3). This suggests that this region, Vβ-SR (for Vβ-specific region in Fig. 3), is tightly involved in interaction with Vβ in determining the Vβ specificity. On one hand, the Vβ-SR has been selectively conserved through evolution of the *Mus* species, preserving the possibility for Mtv to promote stimulation of the host cells. On the other hand, discrete changes in the Vβ-SR may generate new reactivities enlarging the spectrum of interactions. Both mechanisms would contribute to the maintenance and the propagation of the virus.

```
MTV                         Vß-SR                      Vß
                         <---------->
Mtv-DDO      LIHLKVFFNSREEVKKHLIESIKALPLAY            2

                         <---------->
Mtv-1        m--w---Y-----a-R-i--h-------F            3, 17a2
Mtv-3        m--w---Y-----a-R-i--h------TF            3, (17a2?)
Mtv-6        m--w---Y-----a-R-i--h-------F            3, 17a2
Mtv-13       m--w---Y-----a-R-i--h-------F            3, (17a2?)
Mtv-MAI      mK-wR-----KK-aRE-i--h------TV            3, 17a2

Mtv-7        mnfwgki-dyt--gaIak-LynMkythGgrVgfdpf     6, 7, 8.1, 9
MMTV-SW      mnfwgki-dyt--gaIak-IynIkythGgrIgfdpf     6, 7, 8.1, 9
Mtv-43       mnfwgki-dyt--gaVak-LynMkythNgrIgfdpf     6, 7, 8.1, 9

Mtv-8        MnvwGki-hytk gavarQlehisadtfGMSynG       5, 11, 12
Mtv-11       MnvwGki-hytk gavarQlehisadtfGMSynG       11, 12
Mtv-17       InvwKki-hytk gavarQlehisadtfDIRynK       ?
Mtv-9        MnvwGki-hytk gavarLlehisadtfGMSynG       5, 11, 12, 17

MMTV-C3H     mhfwgkI-htk-gTvag---hys-ktygmsyyE        14, 15
MMTV-GR      mhfwgkV-htk-gAvag---hys-ktygmsyyD        14, 15
```

FIGURE 3 Structure of the Mtv region controlling specificity toward Vβ domains. The carboxy-terminal extremity of Mtv-DDO is presented on the top, and the corresponding regions from the other Mtv are aligned below. Mtv regions are grouped according to the Vβ specificities indicated on the right. Question marks indicate unknown or not assessed Vβ target. Dashes stand for amino acid identities, lowercase characters for residues that are Mtv from the same family, and uppercase characters for differences in Mtv of the same family. The Vβ-specific region is indicated by Vβ-SR above the Mtv-DDO and Mtv-1 family. (Mtv-DDO, E. Jouvin-Marche et al., [in prep.]; for the other Mtv we used the corrected sequences from Brandt-Carlson et al. [1993]).

ACKNOWLEDGMENTS

The authors greatly acknowledge D. Voegtlé, C. Liebe-Gris, and J.P. Corre for expert technical assistance, and M. Berson for graphic art works. We are endebted to F. Bonhomme and G.P. Talwar for breeding and generously providing animals. This work was supported by institutional grants from Institut Pasteur, CNRS, and Université Pierre et Marie Curie, and by specific grants from INSERM (no. 920607), Association pour la Recherche sur le Cancer (no. 6692), Ligue de la Recherche sur le Cancer and Fondation pour la Recherche Médicale. A.S. is a recipient of a MRE doctoral fellowship; E.J.-M. and P.N.M. are investigators from the INSERM.

REFERENCES

Abe, R. and R.J. Hodes. 1989. Properties of the Mls system: A revised formulation of Mls genetics and an analysis of T-cell recognition of Mls determinants. *Immunol. Rev.* **107:** 5.

Acha-Orbea, H., A.N. Shakhov, L. Scarpellino, E. Kolb, V. Müller, A. Vessaz-Shaw, R. Fuchs, K. Blöchlinger, P. Rollini, J. Billotte, M. Sarafidou, H.R. MacDonald, and H. Diggelmann. 1991. Clonal deletion of Vβ14-bearing T cells in mice transgenic for mammary tumour virus. *Nature* **350:** 207.

Arden, B., J.L. Klotz, G. Siu, and L.E. Hood. 1985. Diversity and structure of genes of the α family of mouse T cell antigen receptor. *Nature* **316:** 783.

Behlke, M., H. Chou, K. Huppi, and D.Y. Loh. 1986. Murine T cell receptor mutants with deletions of beta-chain variable region genes. *Proc. Natl. Acad. Sci.* **83:** 767.

Bill, J., O. Kanagawa, D.L. Woodland, and E.D. Palmer. 1989. The MHC molecule I-E is necessary but not sufficient for the clonal deletion of Vβ11-bearing T cells. *J. Exp. Med.* **169:** 1405.

Bonhomme, F. and J.L. Guénet. 1989. The wild house mouse and its relatives. In *Genetic variants and strains of the laboratory mouse* (ed. M.F. Lyon and A.G. Searle), p. 649. Gustav Fisher Verlag, Stuttgart.

Brandt-Carlson, C., J.S. Butel, and D. Wheeler. 1993. Phylogenetic and structural analyses of MMTV LTR ORF sequences of exogenous and endogenous origins. *Virology* **193:** 171.

Callahan, R., W. Drohan, D. Gallahan, L. D'Hoostelaere, and M. Potter. 1982. Novel class of mouse mammary tumor virus-related DNA sequences found in all species of *Mus*, including mice lacking the virus proviral genome. *Proc. Natl. Acad. Sci.* **79:** 4113.

Cazenave, P.-A., P.N. Marche, E. Jouvin-Marche, D. Voegtle, F. Bonhomme, A. Bandeira, and A. Coutinho. 1990. Vβ17 gene polymorphism in wild-derived mouse strains: Two amino acid substitutions in the Vβ17 region greatly alter T cell receptor specificity. *Cell* **63:** 717.

Choi, Y., J.W. Kappler, and P. Marrack. 1991. Superantigen encoded in the open reading frame of the 3′ long terminal repeat of mouse mammary tumour virus. *Nature* **350:** 203.

Chou, H.S., C.A. Nelson, S.A. Godambe, D.D. Chaplin, and D.Y. Loh. 1987. Germline organization of the murine T cell receptor β-chain genes. *Science* **238:** 545.

Davis, M.M. and P.J. Bjorkman. 1988. T-cell antigen receptor genes and T-cell recognition. *Nature* **334:** 395.

Dyson, P.J., A. M. Knight, S. Fairchild, E. Simpson, and K. Tomonari. 1991. Genes encoding ligands for deletion of Vβ11 T cells cosegregate with mammary tumour virus genomes. *Nature* **349:** 531.

Frankel, W.N., C. Rudy, J.M. Coffin, and B.T. Huber. 1991. Linkage of *Mls* genes to endogenous mammary tumour viruses of inbred mice. *Nature* **349:** 526.

Haqqi, T.M., S. Banerjee, G.D. Anderson, and C.S. David. 1989. RIII S/J (H-2r). An inbred mouse strain with a massive deletion of T cell receptor Vβ genes. *J. Exp. Med.* **169:** 1903.

Herman, A., J.W. Kappler, P. Marrack, and A.M. Pullen. 1991. Superantigens: Mechanism of T-cell stimulation and role in immune responses. *Annu. Rev. Immunol.* **9:** 745.

Janeway C.A., Jr. 1991. Selective elements for the Vß region of the T cell receptor. *Adv. Immunol.* **50:** 1.

Janeway, C.A., Jr., Y. Yagi, P.J. Conrad, M.E. Katz, B. Jones, S. Vroegop, and S. Buxser. 1989. T cell responses to Mls and to bacterial proteins that mimic its behavior. *Immunol. Rev.* **107:** 61.

Jouvin-Marche, E., P.N. Marche, and P.-A. Cazenave. 1992a. Clonal deletion of Vβ17 T cells in mice from natural populations. *Semin. Immunol.* **4:** 305.

Jouvin-Marche, E., P.-A. Cazenave, D. Voegtlé, and P.N. Marche. 1992b. Vβ17 T-cell deletion by endogenous mammary tumor virus in wild-type-derived mouse strain. *Proc. Natl. Acad. Sci.* **89:** 3232.

Jouvin-Marche, E., N.S. Trede, A. Bandeira, A. Tomas, D.Y. Loh, and P.-A. Cazenave. 1989. Different large deletions of T cell receptor Vβ genes in natural populations of mice. *Eur. J. Immunol.* **19:** 1921.

Kanagawa, O., E. Palmer, and J. Bill. 1989. T cell receptor Vβ6 domain imparts reactivity to the Mls-1[a] antigen. *Cell. Immunol.* **119:** 412.

Kappler, J.W., U. Staerz, J. White, and P.C. Marrack. 1988. Self-tolerance eliminates T cells specific for Mls-modified products of the major histocompatibility complex. *Nature* **332:** 35.

Kappler, J.W., T. Wade, J. White, E. Kushnir, M. Blackman, J. Bill, N. Roehm, and P. Marrack. 1987. A T cell receptor Vβ segment that imparts reactivity to a class II major histocompatibility complex product. *Cell* **49:** 263.

Kozak, C., R. Pauley, V. Morris, R. Michalides, J. Dudley, M. Green, M. Davisson, O. Prakash, A. Vaidra, J. Hilgers, A. Verstraeten, N. Hynes, H. Diggelmann, D. Peterson, J.C. Cohen, C. Dickson, N. Sarkar, R. Nusse, H. Varmus, and R. Callahan. 1987. A standardized nomenclature for endogenous mouse mammary tumor viruses. *J. Virol.* **61:** 651.

Leo, O., M. Foo, D.H. Sachs, L.E. Samelson, and J.A. Bluestone. 1987. Identification of a monoclonal antibody specific for a murine T3 polypeptide. *Proc. Natl. Acad. Sci.* **84:** 1374.

Liao, N.S., J. Maltzman, and D.H. Raulet. 1989. Positive selection determine T cell receptor Vβ14 gene usage by CD8[+] T cells. *J. Exp. Med.* **170:** 135.

Louie, M.C., C.A. Nelson, and D.Y. Loh. 1989. Identification and characterization of new murine T cell receptor β chain Variable region

(Vβ) genes. *J. Exp. Med.* **170:** 1987.

MacDonald, H.R., R. Schneider, R.K. Lees, R.C. Howe, H. Acha-Orbea, H. Festenstein, R. M. Zinkernagel, and H. Hengartner. 1988. T-cell receptor Vβ use predicts reactivity and tolerance to Mls [a]-encoded antigens. *Nature* **332:** 40.

Majors, J.E. and H.E. Varmus. 1983. Nucleotide sequencing of an apparent proviral copy of *env* mRNA defines determinants of expression of the mouse mammary tumor virus *env* gene. *J. Virol.* **47:** 495.

Malissen, M., C. McCoy, D. Blanc, J. Trucy, C. DeVaux, A.M. Schmitt-Verhulst, F. Fitch, L. Hood, and B. Malissen. 1986. Direct evidence for chromosomal inversion during T-cell receptor β-gene rearrangements. *Nature* **319:** 28.

Marrack, P., E. Kushnir, and J. Kappler. 1991. A maternally inherited superantigen encoded by a mammary tumour virus. *Nature* **349:** 524.

Necker, A., N. Rebaï, M. Matthes, E. Jouvin-Marche, P.-A. Cazenave, P. Swarnworawong, E. Palmer, H.R. MacDonald, and B. Malissen. 1991. Monoclonal antibodies raised against engineered soluble mouse T cell receptors and specific for Vα8-, Vβ2- or Vβ10-bearing T cells. *Eur. J. Immunol.* **21:** 3035.

Okada, C.Y., B. Holzmann, S. Guidos, E. Palmer, and I.L. Weissman. 1990. Characterization of a rat antibody specific for a determinant encoded by the Vβ7 gene segment. Depletion of Vβ7[+] T cells in mice with Mls-1[a] haplotype. *J. Immunol.* **144:** 3473.

Pullen, A., P. Marrack, and J. Kappler. 1988. The T-cell repertoire is heavily influenced by tolerance to polymorphic self antigens. *Nature* **335:**796.

Pullen, A.M., W. Potts, E.K. Wakeland, J. Kappler, and P. Marrack. 1990. Surprisingly uneven distribution of the T cell receptor Vβ repertoire in wild mice. *J. Exp. Med.* **171:** 49.

Singer, P.A., R.S. Balderas, and A.N. Theofilopoulos. 1990. Thymic selection defines multiple T cell receptor Vβ "repertoire phenotypes" at the CD4/CD8 subset level. *EMBO J.* **9:** 3641.

Six, A., E. Jouvin-Marche, D.Y. Loh, P.-A. Cazenave, and P.N. Marche. 1991. Identification of a T cell receptor β chain variable region, Vβ20, that is differentially expressed in various strains of mice. *J. Exp. Med.* **174:** 1263.

Tomonari, K., and H. Hengartner. 1992. Positive selection of TCRβ-V10β[+] T cells. *Immunogenetics* **35:** 9.

Tomonari, K., S. Fairchild, and O.A. Rosenwasser. 1993. Influence of viral superantigens on Vβ- and Vα-specific positive and negative selection. *Immunol. Rev.* **131:** 131.

Tomonari, K., E. Lovering, and S. Spencer. 1990. Correlation between the Vβ4[+] CD8[+] T-cell population and the H-2 haplotype. *Immunogenetics* **31:** 333.

Vacchio, M.S., J.J. Ryan, and R.J. Hodes. 1990. Characterization of the ligand(s) responsible for negative of Vβ11- and β12-expressing T cells: Effects of a new Mls determinant. *J. Exp. Med.* **172:** 807.

Wade, T., J. Bill, P.C. Marrack, E. Palmer, and J.W. Kappler. 1988. Molecular basis for the nonexpression of Vβ17 in some strains of mice. *J. Immunol.* **141:** 2165.

White, J., A. Herman, A.M. Pullen, R. Kubo, J. Kappler, and P. Marrack. 1989. The Vβ-specific superantigen staphylococcal enterotoxin B: Stimulation of mature T cells and clonal deletion in neonatal mice. *Cell* **56:** 27.

Woodland, D., M.P. Happ, J. Bill, and E. Palmer. 1990. Requirement for cotolerogenic gene products in the clonal deletion of I-E reactive T cells. *Science* **247:** 964.

Woodland, D.L., M.P. Happ, K.J. Gollob, and E. Palmer. 1991. An endogenous retrovirus mediating deletion of αβ T cells? *Nature* **349:** 529.

T-Cell Recognition of Superantigen: Role of Non-Vβ TCR Elements and MHC Molecules

M.A. Blackman,[1,2] **H.P. Smith,**[1] **R. Wen,**[2]
A.M. Deckhut,[1] **and D.L. Woodland**[1,2]

[1]Department of Immunology, St. Jude Children's Research Hospital, Memphis, Tennessee 38105
[2]Department of Pathology, University of Tennessee, Memphis, Tennessee 38163

Superantigens are characterized by their ability to stimulate families of T cells that share T-cell receptor (TCR) Vβ elements, essentially independently of the other elements of the TCR and polymorphic variation in the major histocompatibility complex (MHC)-presenting molecule (for review, see Herman et al. 1991a). These two unusual characteristics suggested that T-cell recognition of superantigen differed from that described for recognition of conventional antigen/MHC. This idea was quickly supported by experimental data. Several investigators, using both mutagenesis (Cazanave et al. 1990; Choi et al. 1990; Pullen et al. 1990, 1991; Mollick et al. 1993) and peptide inhibition (Pontzer et al. 1992) approaches, showed that the superantigen interacted with residues on the Vβ element predicted to lie on the outer, solvent-exposed face of the molecule, far away from the putative binding site for conventional antigen/MHC. In addition, the MHC-binding site for bacterial superantigen was shown to be on the outside of the molecule, rather than in the peptide-binding cleft (Dellabona et al. 1990; Herman et al. 1991b; Karp and Long 1992). Binding of retroviral superantigen to MHC has yet to be characterized. These studies suggested a model in which the superantigen served as a cross-linking molecule that bridged the T cell and the antigen-presenting cell. However, not all the data were consistent with this model. First, the TCR Vβ element did not absolutely predict superantigen reactivity. Most, but not all, T cells bearing the relevant Vβ element responded to a given superantigen. It was proposed that the few nonreactive cells resulted from a negative contribution of non-Vβ TCR elements which, in rare cases, prevented productive interaction with superantigen (Kappler et al. 1987, 1988). Second, whereas most T cell/superantigen interactions were independent of MHC polymorphism, several examples were reported in which the MHC molecule influenced reactivity of individual T cells for superantigen (Herman et al. 1990; Scholl et al. 1990; Fleischer and Mittrucker 1991; Mollick et al. 1991; Yagi et al. 1991). These data suggested that non-Vβ elements of the TCR and polymorphic regions of the MHC molecule played a role in at least some TCR/superantigen interactions.

ROLE FOR NON-Vβ ELEMENTS OF THE TCR IN SUPERANTIGEN RECOGNITION

Previous attempts to define the non-Vβ TCR contribution to superantigen recognition in a panel of murine Vβ17+ hybridomas were inconclusive, largely because the contribution of Vα, Jα, Dβ, and Jβ could not be analyzed simultaneously in relatively small panels of hybridomas (Kappler et al. 1987; Blackman et al. 1988). Therefore, we have undertaken a reexamination of the question in a Vβ8.1 transgenic mouse model, in which the β chain is invariant, allowing direct assessment of the role of the α chain in recognition of the mouse mammary tumor virus (Mtv) -7-associated superantigen, Mls-1 (Smith et al. 1992). The transgenic β chain, Vβ8.1 Dβ2 Jβ2.3 Cβ2, was cloned from a T-cell hybridoma that was strongly Mls-1-reactive. However, the transgenic T cells were unusually variable in their Mls-1-reactivity, suggesting a possible role of the α chain. For example, only about 50% of Vβ8.1+ thymocytes were clonally deleted in transgenic mice that expressed Mls-1 endogenously (Blackman et al. 1990). To investigate the influence of the α chain, we generated a large panel of T-cell hybridomas from both Mls-1- and Mls-1+ Vβ8.1 transgenic mice and characterized the hybridomas for Mls-1-reactivity and α-chain usage. Only hybridomas that demonstrated strong reactivity to anti-TCR stimulation and expressed a single $V\alpha$ message were included in the panel. A summary of the analysis in Table 1 indicates that there was no direct correlation between $V\alpha$ expression and Mls-1-reactivity. However, biases for or against Mls-1-reactivity were seen. For example, most $V\alpha11^+$ transgenic T cells were Mls-1-reactive, and most $V\alpha2^+$ and $V\alpha8^+$ transgenic hybridomas were not Mls-1-reactive.

To determine whether Mls-1 reactivity within the $V\alpha2^+$ and $V\alpha11^+$ hybridomas segregated with individual family members, and to determine the $J\alpha$ element and junctional diversity, the α chains from these hybridomas were sequenced. The $V\alpha11^+$ hybrids expressed one of two family members, $V\alpha11.1$ and $V\alpha11.3$, and there was a precise correlation between family member and Mls-1 reactivity, in that the seven $V\alpha11.1^+$ hybridomas were all Mls-1-reactive, whereas the two $V\alpha11.3^+$ hybridomas were not (Fig. 1A; Table 2). There was no overlap in $J\alpha$ usage in this small panel (Table 2). In contrast, the $V\alpha2^+$ hybridomas expressed seven different family members, and there was no correlation with Mls-1-reactivity (Fig. 1B; Table 2). There was also no correlation between Mls-1-reactivity and $J\alpha$ usage (Fig. 1C; Table 2). Interestingly, two hybridomas, one strongly Mls-1-reactive and one not reactive, expressed $V\alpha2.3$

TABLE 1 *CORRELATION BETWEEN $V\alpha$ USAGE AND Mls-1 REACTIVITY IN T-CELL HYBRIDOMAS FROM TCR $V\beta8.1$ β-CHAIN TRANSGENIC MICE*

Source of hybridoma	Mls-1 reactivity	$V\alpha$ usage (number of hybridomas)							
		$V\alpha1$	$V\alpha2$	$V\alpha4$	$V\alpha5$	$V\alpha6$	$V\alpha8$	$V\alpha11$	$V\alpha13$
Mls$^-\beta$TG	+	5	3	6	1	3	1	10	1
	−	1	8	9	0	1	10	2	2
Mls$^+\beta$TG	+	0	4	0	0	0	0	0	0
	−	4	12	6	0	1	12	0	2

Hybridomas were generated from Mls-1$^+$ and Mls-1$^-$ Vβ8.1 transgenic mice following stimulation of T cells with KJ16 (anti-Vβ8.1 + Vβ8.2). Mls-1 reactivity is determined by the secretion of IL-2 in response to Mls-1$^+$ spleen cells. All hybridomas in the panel secrete IL-2 in response to stimulation with immobilized anti-Vβ8 antibodies. $V\alpha$ usage was determined by hybridization of hybridoma RNA with a panel of $V\alpha$-specific probes, as described previously (Smith et al. 1992). Only hybridomas that expressed a single $V\alpha$ message were included in the table.

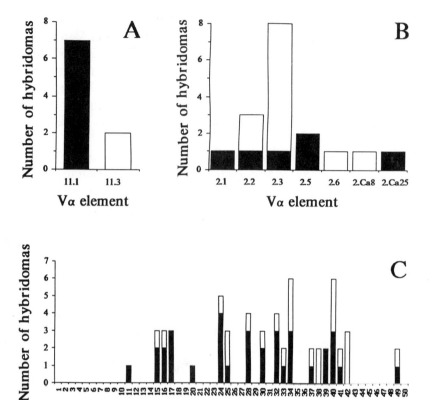

FIGURE 1 Influence of Vα11 family members (A), Vα2 family members (B), and Jα elements (C) on Mls-1 recognition by transgenic Vβ8.1⁺ T-cell hybridomas. The total number of hybridomas in each group is represented as a single bar. The fraction of those hybridomas that are Mls-1-reactive in each group is indicated by the shaded portion of each bar.

and Jα40, with only two amino acid differences in the junction. Site-directed mutagenesis studies are in progress to establish whether the sequence differences in the junction are directly controlling Mls-1 reactivity.

The panel of transgenic hybridomas was also analyzed for reactivity to a bacterial superantigen, staphylococcal enterotoxin B (SEB). The data presented in Table 2 show that, although 23 of 25 hybridomas responded to SEB, there were dif-

TABLE 2 *Vα USAGE AND SUPERANTIGEN REACTIVITY OF INDIVIDUAL Vβ8.1 TRANSGENIC HYBRIDOMAS*

Hybridoma	Vα	Jα	Mls reactivity	SEB reactivity
2–26	11.1	16	+	++
2–47	11.1	7	+	++
2–2	11.1	39	+	++
2–1	11.1	40	+	++
1–34	11.1	33	+	++
4–2	11.1	33	+	++
3–36	11.1	10	+	++
3–5	2.5	24	+	++
1–6	2.2	32	+	–
1–27	2.1	11	+	+
1–24.11	2.3	40	+	++
1–16	2.5	17	+	+
3–25	2.Ca25	16	+	+
3–33	11.3	20	–	+
4–43	11.3	31	–	–
1–23.4	2.3	40	–	+
1–10.2	2.3	41	–	+
1–52.10	2.2	38	–	+
1–43	2.3	25	–	+
1–46	2.3	42	–	+
1–2	2.3	38	–	+
1–4.6	2.3	25	–	+
4–47	2.2	40	–	+
1–10.3	2.6	30	–	++
1–8	2.Ca8	42	–	+

The α chains from Vα11[+] and Vα2[+] Vβ8.1 transgenic T-cell hybridomas were sequenced, as described previously (Smith et al. 1992). Those hybridomas that secreted >10 units/ml IL-2 in response to Mls-1 presented by spleen cells from Mls-1[+] H-2^k, H-2^b, or H-2^d strains of mice are scored as +. SEB-reactive hybridomas are scored as + or ++, based on the concentration of SEB in μg/ml required to give half-maximal stimulation, as described previously (Smith et al. 1992). Hybridomas scored as – for SEB failed to respond at any concentration up to 50 μg/ml.

ferences in the concentration of SEB required for half-maximal stimulation, which correlated with α-chain usage. Thus, Vα11.1$^+$ hybridomas were strongly SEB-reactive, whereas Vα11.3$^+$ hybridomas were weakly reactive or nonreactive. These patterns correlated precisely with the patterns of Mls-1 reactivity. In contrast, the Vα2$^+$ hybridomas demonstrated a more complex pattern. They were heterogeneous for SEB reactivity, and, as for Mls-1 reactivity, there was no apparent correlation with Vα2 family member or Jα. In addition, there was not a direct correlation between Mls-1 reactivity and SEB reactivity of individual hybridomas. For example, the Mls-1-reactive Vα2$^+$ hybridomas exhibited a range of SEB reactivity from none to relatively strong, and one non-Mls-1-reactive hybridoma was strongly SEB-reactive. Thus, the α-chain component of the TCR differentially affected the reactivity of the transgenic hybridomas to two different superantigens.

These data indicate that there is a strong influence of the α chain on Mls-1 and SEB recognition of individual T cells that express the same (transgenic) Vβ8.1$^+$ β chain. Two independent studies have analyzed the α-chain contribution to Mls-1 reactivity of nontransgenic Vβ6$^+$ T cells, using monoclonal antibodies, and have shown a similar bias of Vα2$^+$ T cells *against* and Vα11$^+$ T cells *for* Mls-1 (Vacchio et al. 1992; Waanders et al. 1993). In addition, in agreement with our finding that most Vα2$^+$ transgenic Vβ8.1$^+$ hybridomas are not strongly SEB-reactive, a bias against SEB reactivity has been shown in vivo for Vα2$^+$ transgenic Vβ8.2$^+$ T cells (Waanders et al. 1993). The consistency of the Vα correlations for different Vβs and different superantigens was unexpected, because it indicated a β-chain-independent role of the TCR α chain in superantigen recognition.

INFLUENCE OF THE TCR α CHAIN ON T-CELL TOLERANCE TO Mls-1 IN Vβ8.1 TRANSGENIC MICE

Most Vβ8.1$^+$ T cells are absent from the periphery of Mls-1$^+$ mice, because of efficient thymic clonal deletion. In contrast, we detected incomplete deletion in Mls-1$^+$ Vβ8.1 transgenic mice, and normal numbers of peripheral T cells (Blackman et al. 1990). However, the mouse was tolerant to Mls-1, as measured by lack of in vitro responsiveness, and there was no evidence of overt autoimmune disease. Functional analysis of the $CD4^+V\beta8.1^+$ transgenic T cells showed that up to 50% were anergic, or nonresponsive to stimulation via the TCR (Blackman et al. 1991). We could thus distinguish three groups of T cells in these mice, depending on whether they were clonally deleted, anergized, or unaffected by Mls-1. We hypothesized that the fate of individual transgenic T cells in an Mls-1$^+$ mouse depended on the affinity for Mls-1, determined by the endogenous α chain with which the transgenic β chain had paired. Thus, cells bearing TCR of high affinity for Mls-1 were clonally deleted in the thymus. T cells of intermediate affinity escaped clonal deletion in the thymus but were tolerized in the periphery by mechanisms of anergy or peripheral deletion. Finally, T cells of low (or no) affinity for Mls-1 were unaffected by the presence of Mls-1. The hybridoma frequency analysis (Table 1) supports this hypothesis, in that the bias of $V\alpha11^+$ hybridomas for Mls-1 reactivity and $V\alpha2^+$ and $V\alpha8^+$ hybridomas against Mls-1-reactivity was also reflected in the tolerized repertoire from Mls-1-expressing transgenic mice (Table 1). No $V\alpha11^+$ hybridomas were identified from these mice, indicating that they had been deleted from the functional repertoire. In contrast, the percentage of $V\alpha2^+$ and $V\alpha8^+$ hybridomas increased significantly (from 17% to 39% for $V\alpha2$; from 17% to 29% for $V\alpha8$), as expected if they were relatively less affected by mechanisms of tolerance. We have obtained recent direct evidence to support the conclusion that $V\alpha2^+$ transgenic T cells are relatively less efficiently deleted in the thymus of Mls-1$^+$ mice, accounting, in large part, for their increased frequency in the periphery (data not shown). Thus, the α-chain contribution to superantigen reactivity of individual T cells can have profound effects on their susceptibility to tolerance.

ROLE OF THE MHC MOLECULE IN SUPERANTIGEN RECOGNITION

Although T-cell recognition of superantigen is not classically MHC-restricted, in that most T cells recognize superantigen presented by multiple MHC alleles and isotypes, there is a well-defined heirarchy of presentation. For example, in the mouse, I-E>I-A, and H-2^k>H-2^d>H-2^b>H-2^q. This has been attributed to differences in binding of the superantigen to different class II molecules, rather than TCR specificity. However, infrequent examples of MHC-specific recognition of superantigen by individual clones and hybridomas have been described (Herman et al. 1990; Scholl et al. 1990; Fleischer and Mittrucker 1991; Mollick et al. 1991; Yagi et al. 1991).

Our own studies were prompted by our finding that individual Vβ17$^+$ hybridomas were able to distinguish the Mtv-9-associated superantigen, vSAG-9, presented by H-2^k or H-2^d (Blackman et al. 1992). Some hybridomas recognized vSAG-9 presented only by H-2^k, or presented only by H-2^d, whereas other hybridomas recognized vSAG-9 presented by either H-2^k or H-2^d. The recognition pattern was consistent whether the superantigen was presented by spleen cells isolated from Mtv-9-expressing mice of the appropriate MHC haplotypes, or by IA^{k}IE^k and IA^{d}IE^d B-cell tumor lines that had been stably transfected with vSAG-9. The cross patterns of specificity eliminated the possibility that the results could be explained by differences in the affinity of vSAG-9 for individual class II molecules or by differences in accessory molecules expressed on the hybridomas.

These findings were unexpected, because a strong influence of MHC polymorphisms on Mls-1-reactive T cells had not been described previously. Therefore, in order to determine whether recognition of vSAG-9 by Vβ17$^+$ T cells was unique, and fundamentally different from recognition of Mls-1, we analyzed the influence of MHC on the recognition of vSAG-9 by Vβ17$^+$ and Vβ5$^+$ T-cell hybridomas, and the recognition of Mls-1 by Vβ8.1$^+$ and Vβ8.2$^+$ T-cell hybridomas (Woodland et al. 1993). The results are summarized in Table 3. First, recognition of vSAG-9 by Vβ5$^+$ T-cell hybridomas was also strongly influenced by the MHC haplotype of the presenting cell. Although relatively few hybridomas were superantigen-reactive, the majority of these recognized vSAG-9 exclusively in the context of either H-2^k or H-2^d. Thus, MHC-specific recognition of Mtv-9 was not a characteristic unique to Vβ17$^+$ T cells. Second, a strong influence of the specificity of the MHC-pre-

TABLE 3 *MHC SPECIFICITY OF SUPERANTIGEN RECOGNITION*

Vβ	vSAG	Number of hybrids	% of hybridomas recognizing superantigen presented by different MHC haplotypes			
			$H\text{-}2^k$	$H\text{-}2^d$	$H\text{-}2^k + H\text{-}2^d$	neither $H\text{-}2^k$ nor $H\text{-}2^d$
5	9	96	18	8	16	58
17	9	90	11	16	52	21
8.1	7	17	6	0	94	0
8.2	7	31	16	6	16	62
TG Vβ8.1	7	73	29	0	53	18
TG Vα2Vβ8.1	7	43	51	2	5	42

MHC-specific recognition of retroviral superantigens by T-cell hybridomas. T-cell hybridomas bearing different Vβ elements were generated by fusing T cells responding to immobilized anti-Vβ antibodies with BW5147, as described previously (Woodland et al. 1993). Superantigen reactivity was determined by assessing IL-2 secretion in response to vSAG-7 or vSAG-9 presented on transfectants and/or spleen cells. Nonreactive hybridomas did not respond to superantigen presented by H-2^k or H-2^d, although they did secrete IL-2 in response to immobilized anti-Vβ antibody.

senting molecule was seen in the recognition of Mls-1 by Vβ8.2+ T-cell hybridomas, in that 7 of 12 distinguished Mls-1 presented by H-2^k and H-2^d. Thus, there appeared to be no fundamental difference between recognition of Mls-1 and vSAG-9. Third, 16 of 17 Vβ8.1+ hybridomas recognized Mls-1 regardless of the haplotype of the presenting molecule, consistent with previous data that showed no evidence for MHC specificity in T-cell recognition of Mls-1 by Vβ8.1+ T cells (Peck et al. 1977; DeKruyff et al. 1986; Kappler et al. 1988). This difference in Mls-1 recognition by Vβ8.1+ and Vβ8.2+ T cells is discussed below.

We also examined the role of the MHC molecule in Mls-1 recognition by the Vβ8.1 transgenic hybridomas described earlier. In striking contrast to non-transgenic Vβ8.1+ T cells, a significant percentage of the transgenic hybridomas demonstrated MHC-specific recognition of Mls-1. Not only were the transgenic Vβ8.1 hybridomas more MHC-specific in their Mls-1 reactivity, but also a significant percentage of them exhibited an unusual MHC-specificity pattern, in that they recognized Mls-1 presented by H-2^k and/or H-2^b, but not H-2^d. Normally H-2^d is a strong presenter of Mls-1 to Vβ8.1+ T cells (Kappler et al. 1988). Using a monoclonal antibody (Pircher et al. 1992) to identify the subset of Vα2+ transgenic Vβ8.1+ hybridomas, we found that virtually all of them fell within this group of unusual MHC specificity (Woodland et al. 1993).

CORRELATION OF THE TCR α CHAIN WITH MHC-SPECIFIC RECOGNITION OF Mls-1

By using a Vβ8.1 transgenic mouse to fix the β chain, we have revealed a role for the α chain in Mls-1 recognition (see above) and also defined an influence of the MHC-haplotype on the interaction. Sequence analysis of the α chain of the Vα2+ transgenic Vβ8.1 hybridomas was carried out in an attempt to correlate sequence motifs with the patterns of MHC bias demonstrated by this structurally homogeneous group of T cells (Woodland et al. 1993). Altogether, 29 Vα2+ α chains were sequenced. There was no direct correlation between Vα2 family member or Jα usage and pattern of MHC bias (data not shown). However, the Jα usage was not completely overlapping, which may indicate that Jα plays a role (Fig. 2). No patterns of junctional diversity emerged from the analysis, but two hybridomas, one of which recognized Mls-1 in the context of H-2^k only and the other in the context of H-2^b only, used the same Vα2 family member (2.3) and the same Jα (39), and differed in the two junctional amino acids, strongly implicating the junctional region in MHC specificity of superantigen recognition. Thus, although this analysis cannot establish general rules for the α-chain contribution to Mls-1 reactivity, both the correlation established above for Mls-1 reactivity and non-reactivity (Smith et al. 1992), and the correlation established here for MHC specificity (Woodland et al. 1993), implicate junctional amino acids.

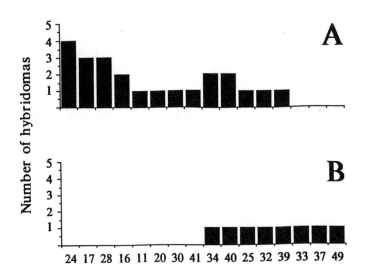

Jα-element

FIGURE 2 Influence of Jα elements on the MHC-specific recognition of Mls-1 by transgenic Vβ8.1$^+$ T-cell hybridomas. Jα usage of hybridomas that preferentially recognized Mls-1 in the context of H-2^k are shown in *A*. Jα usage of hybridomas that preferentially recognize Mls-1 in the context of H-2^b are shown in *B*.

A UNIFYING HYPOTHESIS

Our data indicate that the recognition of superantigens by T cells is more complex than had originally been described. First, we have shown that superantigen reactivity of individual T cells can be influenced both by the Vβ element expressed and by non-Vβ elements of the TCR. Second, we have identified a critical role for polymorphic residues of MHC molecules in the interaction.

We have interpreted these data in the context of a model for T-cell recognition of superantigen in which the TCR and MHC are brought into intimate contact. This has been previously proposed (Janeway et al. 1989) and has been recently supported both by structural data (Swaminathan et al. 1992) and by functional and binding analysis of SEB mutants (Kappler et al. 1992). In some cases, the interaction of the TCR with the MHC is of no consequence, because the affinity of the superantigen for both TCR and MHC is strong. However, when the superantigen has a relatively weak affinity for the MHC or Vβ, the TCR/MHC contacts can make an important contribution to the stability of the trimolecular complex. Thus, the interactions of non-Vβ elements of the TCR with polymorphic residues on the MHC molecule result in MHC specificity.

In this context, the involvement of non-Vβ elements of the TCR and polymorphic residues of the MHC in superantigen recognition is consistent with an inherently low affinity for superantigen. Thus, the differences in recognition of Mls-1 by nontransgenic Vβ8.1[+] T cells, transgenic Vβ8.1[+] T cells, and nontransgenic Vβ8.2[+] T cells may be explained by overall affinity differences. Indirect evidence suggests that Vβ8.1[+] T cells have relatively strong affinity for Mls-1, in that they are easily activated in vitro with Mls-1 and are efficiently clonally deleted in the thymus of Mls-1[+] mice. In contrast, the interaction between Vβ8.2[+] TCR and Mls-1 appears to be relatively weaker (Kappler et al. 1988; Pullen et al. 1991). Similarly, we think that the transgenic β chain is inherently weakly Mls-1-reactive, presumably because of the non-Vβ components of the β chain, and is therefore strongly influenced by the α chain with which it has paired. Thus, in both cases involving (putative) weak Mls-1 interaction, Mls-1 recognition is strongly influenced by non-Vβ elements of the TCR and by polymorphic differences in the MHC molecule.

On the basis of this affinity argument, we would predict an inverse correlation between absolute frequency of super-antigen reactivity (as a measure of the degree of influence of non-Vβ contributions) and degree of MHC specificity. In the limited analysis we have done so far, this correlation holds (Fig. 3). For example, all of the nontransgenic Vβ8.1[+] hybridomas were reactive with Mls-1, and there was no obvious influence of MHC polymorphism on this reactivity. In contrast, only 39% of Vβ8.2[+] hybridomas were Mls-1-reactive, and there was a strong influence of the MHC haplotype of the presenting cell on recognition by individual hybridomas. We would also predict a concordance between CD4 dependency and MHC specificity of superantigen recognition by individual TCR of low inherent avidity for superantigen. Our preliminary results indicate this to be the case (data not shown). A third prediction is that recognition of bacterial toxins, which are stronger superantigens, is unlikely to be MHC-specific. Our data show this to be the case (Blackman et al. 1992), although we have recently identified hybridomas that show MHC-specific recognition of SEB (data not shown).

Our sequence analysis implicates junctional amino acids in MHC-specific superantigen reactivity. This is consistent with an important interaction between MHC or peptide/MHC being controlled by the third hypervariable region of the TCR. In addition, the precise correlation with Vα11.1[+] α chains in the transgenic hybridomas, and the general bias of Vα11[+] Vβ6[+] nontransgenic T cells to Mls-1 reactivity described in two independent studies (Vacchio et al. 1992; Waanders et al. 1993), may reflect the general bias of Vα11[+] α chains for MHC class II, in particular I-E, that has previously suggested (Jameson et al. 1991). Although the most likely contribution of non-Vβ elements of the TCR to superantigen recognition is via direct interaction with the MHC or peptide/MHC, this model does not rule out additional direct interactions between non-Vβ elements of the TCR and superantigen or conformational changes affecting the Vβ/superantigen interaction. In addition, there is no requirement for the proposed interaction between TCR and MHC to be the same as during recognition of conven-

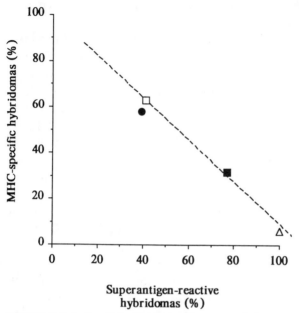

FIGURE 3 Relationship between the overall frequency of superantigen recognition and the frequency of MHC-specific superantigen recognition among different panels of T-cell hybridomas. Four different panels of hybridomas are represented: $V\beta5^+$ (*open box*) and $V\beta17^+$ (*filled box*) hybridomas recognizing vSAG-9; $V\beta8.1^+$ (*open triangle*) and $V\beta8.2^+$ (*filled circle*) hybridomas recognizing Mls-1. The transgenic hybridomas shown in Table 3 are not represented here because they expressed highly biased MHC-specificity patterns in their recognition of Mls-1 due to restriction of the TCR to a single β chain. The percentage of superantigen-reactive hybridomas (x axis) is based on the number of hybridomas that recognize vSAG-9 or Mls-1 in the context of H-2^k and/or H-2^d. Nonreactive hybridomas are defined by their failure to recognize the relevant superantigen even though they express high levels of TCR and CD4, and secrete IL-2 in response to immobilized anti-TCR antibodies. The percentage of MHC-specific hybridomas (y axis) is based on the number of hybridomas that recognize the relevant superantigen exclusively in the context of either H-2^k or H-2^d, compared to the total number of hybridomas that recognize superantigen in the context of either H-2^k and/or H-2^d.

tional antigen/MHC, and there is no requirement for these interactions to be the same for a given T cell with two different superantigens. The molecular nature of the interactions can be addressed by mutagenesis experiments, but a definitive answer may have to await cocrystallization of TCR/superantigen/MHC complexes.

SIGNIFICANCE

The data discussed in this paper show that the Vβ element does not solely determine superantigen reactivity, but that there are contributions both from non-Vβ elements of the TCR and the MHC molecule which, in the case of weak Vβ/superantigen (and/or weak MHC/superantigen) interactions, are required for reactivity. Thus, the distinction between superantigen and conventional antigen may not be as sharp as suggested by the early data because, in many cases, non-Vβ elements of the TCR and specific interaction with MHC may play a critical role. If human viruses contain superantigens, they may be of this weak type and thus show HLA associations and not affect all T cells expressing the implicated Vβ because of the requirement for non-Vβ contributions to the recognition. This may explain why the identification of human viral superantigens, if they exist, has been so elusive.

ACKNOWLEDGMENTS

We thank Phuong Le, Sherri Surman, Twala Hogg, Betsy Sidell, and Jim Houston for excellent technical assistance. This work was supported by National Institutes of Health grants CA-56570, CA-21765, and AI-31489; a Bristol-Myers Cancer Grant Award; and the American Lebanese Syrian Associated Charities (ALSAC).

REFERENCES

Blackman, M.A., J.W. Kappler, and P. Marrack. 1988. T cell specificity and repertoire. *Immunol. Rev.* **101:** 5.

Blackman, M.A., T.H. Finkel, J. Kappler, J. Cambier, and P. Marrack. 1991. Altered antigen receptor signalling in anergic T cells from self-tolerant T-cell receptor β-chain transgenic mice. *Proc. Natl. Acad. Sci.* **88:** 6682.

Blackman, M.A., F.E. Lund, S. Surman, R.B. Corley, and D.L. Woodland. 1992. Major histocompatibility complex-restricted recognition of retroviral superantigens by Vβ17⁺ T cells. *J. Exp. Med.* **176:** 275.

Blackman, M.A., H.-G. Burgert, D.L. Woodland, E. Palmer, J.W. Kappler, and P. Marrack. 1990. A role for clonal inactivation in T cell tolerance to Mls-1ᵃ. *Nature* **345:** 540.

Cazanave, P.-A., P.N. Marche, E. Jouvin-Marche, D. Voegtle, F. Bonhomme, A. Bandeira, and A. Coutinho. 1990. Vβ17 gene polymorphism in wild-derived mouse strains: two amino acid substitutions in the Vβ17 region greatly alter T cell receptor specificity. *Cell* **63:** 717.

Choi, Y., A. Herman, D. DiGiusto, T. Wade, P. Marrack, and J. Kappler. 1990. Residues of the variable region of the T-cell-receptor β-chain that interact with *S. aureus* toxin superantigens. *Nature* **346:** 471.

DeKruyff, R., S. Ju, J. Laning, H. Cantor, and M. Dorf. 1986. Activation requirements of cloned inducer T cells. III. Need for two stimulator cells in the response of a cloned line to Mls determinants. *J. Immunol.* **137:** 1109.

Dellabona, P., J. Peccoud, J. Kappler, P. Marrack, C. Benoist, and D. Mathis. 1990. Superantigens interact with MHC class II molecules outside of the antigen groove. *Cell* **62:** 1115.

Fleischer, B. and H.-W. Mittrucker. 1991. Evidence for T cell receptor-HLA class II molecule interaction in the response to superantigenic bacterial toxins. *Eur. J. Immunol.* **21:** 1331.

Herman, A., J.W. Kappler, P. Marrack, and A.M. Pullen. 1991a. Superantigens: Mechanism of T-cell stimulation and role in immune responses. *Annu. Rev. Immunol.* **9:** 745.

Herman, A., G. Croteau, R.-P. Sekaly, J. Kappler, and P. Marrack. 1990. HLA-DR alleles differ in their ability to present staphylococcal enterotoxins to T cells. *J. Exp. Med.* **172:** 709.

Herman, A., N. Labrecque, J. Thibodeau, P. Marrack, J. Kappler, and R.-P. Sekaly. 1991b. Identification of the staphylococcal enterotoxin A superantigen binding site in the β1 domain of the human histocompatibility antigen HLA-DR. *Proc. Natl. Acad. Sci.* **88:** 9954.

Jameson, S.C., P.B. Nakajima, J.L. Brooks, W. Heath, O. Kanagawa, and N.R.J. Gascoigne. 1991. The T cell receptor Vα11 gene family. Analysis of allelic sequence polymorphism and demonstration of Jα region-dependent recognition by allele-specific antibodies. *J. Immunol.* **147:** 3185.

Janeway, C.A., Jr., J. Yagi, P.J. Conrad, M.E. Katz, B. Jones, S. Vroegop, and S. Buxser. 1989. T-cell responses to Mls and to bacterial proteins that mimic its behavior. *Immunol. Rev.* **107:** 61.

Kappler, J.W., A. Herman, J. Clements, and P. Marrack. 1992. Mutations defining functional regions of the superantigen staphylococcal enterotoxin B. *J. Exp. Med.* 175:387.

Kappler, J.W., U. Staerz, J. White, and P. Marrack. 1988. Self-tolerance eliminates T cells specific for Mls-modified products of the major histocompatibility complex. *Nature* **332:** 35.

Kappler, J.W., T. Wade, J. White, E. Kushnir, M. Blackman, J. Bill, N. Roehm, and P. Marrack. 1987. A T cell reeceptor Vβ segment that imparts reactivity to a class II major histocompatibility complex product. *Cell* **49:** 263.

Karp, D. R. and E.O. Long. 1992. Identification of HLA-DR1 β chain residues critical for binding staphylococcal enterotoxins A and E. *J. Exp. Med.* **175:** 415.

Mollick, J.A., M. Chintagumpala, R.G. Cook, and R.R. Rich. 1991. Staphylococcal exotoxin activation of T cells. Role of exotoxin-MHC class II binding affinity and class II isotype. *J. Immunol.* **146:** 463.

Mollick, J.A., R.L. McMasters, D. Grossman, and R.R. Rich. 1993. Localization of a site on bacterial superantigens that determines T cell receptor β chain specificity. *J. Exp. Med.* **177:** 283.

Peck, A.B., C.A. Janeway, Jr., and H. Wigzell. 1977. T lymphocyte responses to Mls locus antigens involve recognition of I region gene products. *Nature* **266:** 840.

Pircher, H., N. Rebai, M. Groettrup, C. Gregoire, D.E. Speiser, M.P. Happ, E. Palmer, R. Zinkernagel, H. Hengartner, and B. Malissen. 1992. Preferential positive selection of $V\alpha2^+CD8^+$ T cells in mouse strains expressing both $H-2^k$ and T cell receptor $V\alpha^a$ haplotypes: Determination with a Vα2-specific monoclonal antibody. *Eur. J. Immunol.* **22:** 399.

Pontzer, C.M., J. Irwin, N.R.J. Gascoigne, and H.M. Johnson. 1992. T-cell antigen receptor binding sites for the microbial superantigen staphylococcal enterotoxin A. *Proc. Natl. Acad. Sci.* **89:** 7727.

Pullen, A.M., T. Wade, P. Marrack, and J.W. Kappler. 1990. Identification of the region of the T cell receptor β chain that interacts with the self superantigen Mls-1^a. *Cell* **61:**1365.

Pullen, A.M., J. Bill, R.T. Kubo, P. Marrack, and J.W Kappler. 1991. Analysis of the interaction site for the self superantigen Mls-1^a on T cell receptor Vβ. *J. Exp. Med.* **173:** 1183.

Scholl, P.R., A. Diez, R. Karr, R.-P. Sekaly, J. Trowsdale, and R.S. Geha. 1990. Effects of isotypes and allelic polymorphism on the binding of staphylococcal exotoxins to MHC class II molecules. *J. Immunol.* **144:** 226.

Smith, H., P. Le, D.L. Woodland, and M.A. Blackman. 1992. T cell receptor α-chain influences reactivity to Mls-1 in Vβ8.1 transgenic mice. *J. Immunol.* **149:** 887.

Swaminathan, S.W. Furey, J. Pletcher, and M. Sax. 1992. The crystal structure of staphylococcal enterotoxin B, a superantigen. *Nature* **359:** 801.

Vacchio, M.S., O. Kanagawa, K. Tomonari, and R.J. Hodes. 1992. Influence of the T cell receptor Vα expression on Mls^a superantigen-specific T cell responses. *J. Exp. Med.* **175:** 1405.

Woodland, D.L., H.P. Smith, S. Surman, P. Le, R. Wen, and M.A. Blackman. 1993. Major histocompatibility complex-specific recognition of Mls-1 is mediated by multiple elements of the T cell receptor. *J. Exp. Med.* **177:** 433.

Waanders, G.A., A.R. Lussow, and H.R. MacDonald. 1993. Skewed T cell receptor Vα repertoire among superantigen reactive murine T cells. *Int. Immunol.* **5:** 55.

Yagi, J., S. Rath, and C.A. Janeway, Jr. 1991. Control of T cell responses to staphylococcal enterotoxins by stimulator cell MHC class II polymorphism. *J. Immunol.* **147:** 1398.

MTV-encoded Superantigen Expression in B Lymphoma Cells in SJL Mice as a Stimulus for "Reversed Immunological Surveillance"

V.K. Tsiagbe, J. Asakawa,[1] T. Yoshimoto,[2] S.Y. Cho, D. Meruelo, and G.J. Thorbecke

Department of Pathology and Kaplan Cancer Center, New York University School of Medicine, New York, New York 10016

The spontaneously arising SJL follicular center lymphomas (RCS) depend on the cytokine products of host CD4$^+$ T cells, responding to the superantigen-like stimulation by RCS cells, for their growth. All RCS-specific T hybridomas use Vβ16 in their T-cell receptors (TCR), irrespective of what Vα is used in conjunction, and transcription of Vβ16 is specifically increased when polyclonal SJL CD4$^+$ T cells respond to RCS. Extraordinarily high expression of a 1.8-kb mRNA for mouse mammary tumor virus long terminal repeat (MMTV-LTR) was found in both primary lymphomas and in in vitro RCS lines, but not in an SJL B-cell lymphoma, NJ101, that does not stimulate syngeneic T cells or in lipopolysaccharide (LPS)-activated SJL B cells. The cDNA coding for this LTR has been cloned from cRCS-2 and sequenced. Antisense S-oligonucleotides prepared according to 19-mer sequences of the first two potential translation initiation sites of both RCS-*Mtv* and *Mtv-8* reduce the T-cell-stimulating ability of RCS cells. Furthermore, transfection of NJ101 cells with the cloned RCS-MMTV cDNA renders these cells stimulatory for Vβ16 T cells, thus identifying this MMTV-LTR as the coding gene for a superantigen expressed by RCS.

Present addresses: [1]Department of Rheumatology, Juntendo University School of Medicine, Tokyo, Japan; [2]Department of Allergology, Institute of Medical Science, University of Tokyo, Japan.

An oligonucleotide probe prepared according to the 3′ end of this LTR hybridizes with the 1.8-kb mRNA in all RCS tumors, whereas a similar probe made according to the 3′ sequence of *Mtv-8* hybridizes with the larger size RNA present in RCS, NJ101, and normal SJL B cells. Thus, in the SJL lymphoma model, this MMTV serves as a novel oncogene, stimulating lymphoma growth in an indirect T-cell-dependent fashion.

HOST-LYMPHOMA RELATIONSHIP IN THE SJL MOUSE

Virtually all SJL mice develop paraproteinemia of IgG and/or IgA isotypes (Tsiagbe and Thorbecke 1990) and B-cell lymphomas, which are thought to arise in germinal centers (Siegler and Rich 1968) within the first year of life. These lymphomas, called RCS, have several properties that make them resemble human germinal center lymphomas and distinguish them from other murine B-cell lymphomas (Pattengale and Taylor 1983). They exhibit rearranged Ig genes, both of the H and L Ig chains; have deleted μ; and have rearranged J to other isotypes (Stavnezer et al. 1989), but rarely exhibit sIg. Interestingly, they fail to grow in γ-irradiated (Lerman et al. 1976) or athymic (Katz et al. 1981) SJL mice, except when normal SJL lymphoid cells (Lerman et al. 1976) are simultaneously injected. They also do not grow in vitro, unless γ-irradiated SJL lymph node (LN) cells and/or cytokines such as IL-5 and IFN-γ are added (Lasky et al. 1988; Lasky and Thorbecke 1989). This dependence on normal syngeneic T cells for their growth is explained by a process, dubbed "reversed immunological surveillance," that consists of a strong stimulating effect on syngeneic T cells, exerted by all primary RCS (Ponzio et al. 1986), long-transplanted in vivo RCS lines (Lerman et al. 1976; Ponzio et al. 1977a), and tissue-culture cRCS lines (Lasky et al. 1988), and is accompanied by the production in the responding T cells of several cytokines (Hayama et al. 1984; Ponzio et al. 1984; Lasky et al. 1988).

The syngeneic T-cell response to RCS is inhibited by anti-I-A^s and by anti-CD4 (Brown et al. 1983; Ponzio et al. 1987). The properties of this response with respect to magnitude and expression in neonatal SJL thymus (Ponzio et al. 1978) suggest that this is a response to a superantigen, resembling that to *Mls*-like determinants. Other workers have recently shown that most *Mls* and *Mls*-like determinants in mice are closely linked to endogenous MMTV proviral loci (Acha-Orbea et al. 1991; Choi et al. 1991; Dyson et al. 1991; Frankel et al. 1991; Woodland et al. 1991). The product(s) of these loci is implicated in the stimulation of T cells bearing particular TCR Vβ (Choi et al. 1991). More than 30 different endogenous MMTVs have now been mapped and characterized (Kozak et al. 1987). They show about 95% nucleotide sequence homology, with 2–8 different MMTV copies present in the genome of most inbred laboratory mouse strains (Held et al. 1992). MMTV can be expressed in some B-cell lines and in activated normal B cells (Tax et al. 1983; Lopez et al. 1985; King et al. 1990; Lund and Corley 1991). This B-cell expression agrees with the previous observation that *Mls* locus antigens are primarily expressed on B cells (Molina et al. 1989). The results summarized in this paper show that transcription of a novel MMTV provirus in RCS cells confers the superantigen-like properties onto these cells.

FUNCTIONAL PROPERTIES OF RCS-RESPONSIVE T CELLS

The proliferative response of unsensitized syngeneic SJL T to RCS cells is primarily due to CD4$^+$ T cells. Cytotoxic CD8$^+$ T cells are not activated to any significant extent (Ponzio et al. 1977b) and proliferative responses are, if anything, higher when CD8$^+$ T cells are removed (Lerman et al. 1979). To understand the basis of this response, a panel of 21 T hybridomas was generated by fusion of RCS-responding SJL T cells with an αβ TCR-negative variant of BW5147. All of the cloned hybridomas produced IL-2 in response to stimulation with cRCS-X and cRCS-2, and 17 of 21 produced detectable IL-5. There was induction of mRNA for IL-2, IL-4, and IL-5 in RCS-specific hybridomas responding to RCS (not shown). None produced cytokines in response to normal or LPS-activated SJL or (SJL x BALB/c)F$_1$ spleen cells. Responses of RCS-specific T-cell hybridomas to RCS could be inhibited by anti-

I-A^s (Tsiagbe et al. 1993a). A different I-A^s bearing μ^+ B-cell lymphoma (NJ101), derived from an anti-CD4-treated aged SJL mouse (Lin et al. 1992), was not stimulatory for syngeneic T cells or for RCS-specific hybridomas (Fig. 1).

Since RCS-specific T-hybridoma cells produce a variety of cytokines in response to RCS, it was considered of interest to determine whether, like normal SJL LN cells (Lerman et al. 1976), they could promote in vivo growth of RCS in SJL mice that had been γ-irradiated (740 rads) 24 hours before injection of transplantable RCS-X cells. T-hybridoma cells (selected on the basis of high IL-5 production in response to RCS cells), injected alone, did not cause any enlargement of spleen or LN in γ-irradiated SJL mice. Mice receiving RCS-X as well as the T-hybridoma cells showed significantly better growth in both spleen and LN than did mice receiving RCS-X alone (Fig. 2).

PREDOMINANCE OF Vβ16 IN THE RESPONSE TO RCS

Whereas all the RCS-specific T hybridomas stained for CD3, CD4, and $\alpha\beta$ determinants, none of them stained for any of the Vβ TCR determinants to which antibodies were available (Vβ2, -3, -6, -7, -14, and -17a). When blots of total RNA from these hybridomas were hybridized with cDNA probes for Vβ1, -4, -10, -15, -16, and -17, it became quite clear that all the 21 hybridomas bore Vβ16 TCR (Fig. 2) (Tsiagbe et al. 1993a). Preliminary characterization of the two most extensively studied RCS-specific hybridomas by staining for Vα2 TCR expression showed that 1D1-E7 was positive, and 7C5-G4 was negative. In view of previous findings by other investigators (Katz et al. 1988) suggesting that RCS-responsive cells were predominantly Vβ17a$^+$, we included in our experiments a keyhole limpet hemocyanin (KLH)-specific, Vβ17$^+$ hybridoma (SK23-7.4) for staining as well as for probing. In each case, the KLH-specific hybridoma cells were confirmed to be positive, whereas all the 21 RCS-specific hybridomas were found to be negative for Vβ17.

Serial dilutions of RNA samples from SJL LN cells, responding to Con-A or to RCS, were compared with respect to the presence of the relative amounts of mRNA for Vβ1, -4, -10,

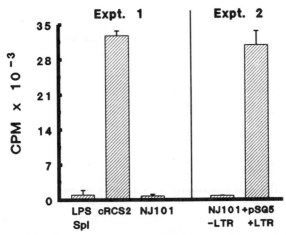

FIGURE 1 Responsiveness of RCS-specific T-hybridoma (1D1-E7) cells to stimulation as measured by [^{3}H]TdR incorporation of 10^4 IL-2-dependent (CTLL-1) cells. (*Expt. 1*) 2 x 10^5 LPS-activated SJL γ-irradiated splenic B cells (LPS Spl., 3000 rads), 2 x 10^4 cRCS-2 cells (9000 rads), or 10^5 NJ101 cells (7000 rads) were used to stimulate 2 x 10^4 hybridoma cells. (*Expt. 2*), 10^5 hybridoma cells were stimulated with 10^5 NJ101 cells (7000 rads), 2 days post-transient transfection with pSG5 plasmid alone or pSG5 containing RCS-*Mtv* LTR.

-15, -16, and -17 by dot blot hybridization. As compared to Con-A stimulation, RCS stimulation resulted in a relatively higher content of mRNA for Vβ16; this was not observed for any of the other Vβs (Tsiagbe et al. 1993a).

As found in previous studies, LN cells from (SJL x BALB/c) F_1 hybrids fail to respond to RCS (Katz et al. 1980), whereas LN cells from SJL mice (4th–6th backcross) transgenic for I-E usually respond well (Tsiagbe et al. 1991). The possibility that Vβ16$^+$ T-cell deletion was more marked in peripheral LN from (SJL x BALB/c) F_1 mice than in LN from I-E$^+$ transgenic SJL mice was therefore examined. As shown in Figure 3B, Vβ17 mRNA was much more prominent in RNA extracted from SJL LN than in RNA from LN of either the F_1 or the I-E$^+$ transgenic mice. I-E$^-$ littermates from the transgenic mice were similar to SJL mice in this respect. In contrast, Vβ16 mRNA was well represented in RNA from LN of SJL, I-E$^+$ transgenic SJL mice and their littermates (8th backcross), whereas very little was seen in the RNA from LN of the F_1 hybrid mice. Thus, respon-

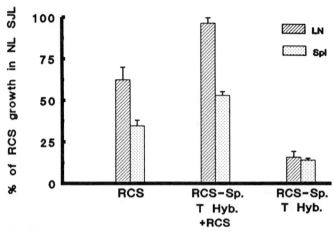

FIGURE 2 Promotion of RCS-X growth by RCS-specific T-hybridoma (1D1-E7) cells in SJL mice, γ-irradiated (740 rads) 2 days prior to injection of RCS-X and hybridoma cells. RCS-specific hybridoma cells (RCS-Sp T Hyb.) were preactivated in vitro for 4 hr with cRCS-2 cells (13,000 rads). 2 x 10^7 T-hybridoma cells were injected i.v. alone or with 5 x 10^6 RCS-X cells (RCS). The LN (brachial, axillary + mesenteric) and spleen weights, 6 days post-injection, were expressed as a percentage of body weight of individual mice (5–7 mice per group). In mice receiving RCS-X as well as the T-hybridoma cells, better RCS growth in spleen (p <0.001) and LN (p <0.005) was obtained than with RCS-X alone. KLH-specific I-A^s-restricted hybridoma (SK24-7.6) cells had no effect on RCS growth even when preactivated in vitro with 5 μg/ml KLH (not shown).

siveness to RCS correlates with expression of Vβ16, and not Vβ17, in peripheral lymphoid tissue of these mice.

COMPARISON OF RCS-SPECIFIC HYBRIDOMAS TO OTHER HYBRIDOMAS

The alloreactive T-cell hybridoma, 3D0-54.8 (bearing Vβ8.3 TCR), which was known to respond to I-A^s (Shimonkevitz et al. 1983), responded to γ-irradiated RCS to a similar extent as did the RCS-specific hybridomas (Table 1). In contrast, the Vβ17a-bearing KLH-specific hybridoma failed to respond to RCS, as did the heme-specific, Vβ1$^+$ T-cell hybridoma. Three CD4$^+$Vα8$^+$Vβ16$^+$ T-cell hybridomas of unknown specificity (kindly donated by Dr. E. Palmer) were also analyzed for reactivity to RCS. All three of these responded with IL-2 production

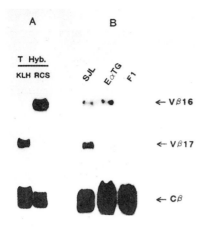

FIGURE 3 Expression of mRNA for Vβ16, Vβ17, and Cβ. (*A*): A KLH-specific I-A^s-restricted hybridoma (SK23-7.4) is compared to an RCS-specific hybridoma (1D1-E7). Similar hybridization patterns were observed for all of 21 RCS-specific hybridomas. (*B*) LN of SJL, I-Eα transgene$^+$ SJL, and (SJL x AKR) F$_1$ mice are compared.

(Tsiagbe et al. 1993a). These findings show that responsiveness of T hybridomas to RCS is determined by the presence of Vβ16 TCR, independent of the MHC class II origin of the T hybridoma and probably also of the Vα TCR subset.

ANTIGEN-PRESENTING PROPERTIES OF RCS CELLS FOR Vβ16⁻ T HYBRIDOMAS

We next determined whether RCS cells could be used as antigen-presenting cells (APC) in the stimulation of antigen-specific hybridomas bearing Vβ other than Vβ16. RCS cells presented heme to BST1-19.3 even when as few as 6 x 10^3 cells were added and were, therefore, much more efficient as APC than whole spleen cells (Tsiagbe et al. 1993a). Since the I-A^s-dependent stimulation of these hybridomas might be the result of an RCS-specific peptide presented by I-A^s, we attempted to block the stimulation of RCS-specific T-hybridoma cells by RCS with an oligopeptide known to bind to I-A^s in a conventional manner (KM core peptide, Lamont et al. 1990) and with a nonprotein I-A^s binder, heme (Cooper et al. 1988).

TABLE 1 REACTIVITY OF Vβ16⁺ HYBRIDOMAS TO RCS

Cell line	Specificity	Vβ	Vα	Response to	
				RCS	RCS + Ag
1D1-E7	RCS	16	2	+	n.d.
7C5-G4	RCS	16	(Vα2⁻)	+	n.d.
4BR181	?	16	8	+	n.d.
3HB100	?	16	8	+	n.d.
3Q19	?	16	8	+	n.d.
3D0-54.8	I-A^d, I-A^s	8.3	n.d.	+	n.d.
SK23-7.4	KLH + I-A^s	17a	n.d.	–	+
BST 1-19.3	heme + I-A^s	1	n.d.	–	+

Derived from Tsiagbe et al. (1993a). n.d. indicates not done.

No inhibition was seen, even though the stimulating RCS cells had been preincubated with 40 μM of KM core peptide for 2 hours, in the presence of protease inhibitors, or with 20 μM heme for 1–2 days prior to stimulation of the hybridoma cells. It should be noted that the concentration of KM core peptide used was 10 times that reported by Lamont et al. (1990) to be needed for 75% inhibition of I-A^s-restricted antigen (Ag) presentation. Thus, even though RCS cells are excellent APC, there is no evidence that conventional RCS-specific peptide presentation is involved in the stimulation of RCS-specific T cells by RCS.

TRANSCRIPT OF MMTV-LTR IN RCS

The possibility that the transcription of a novel MMTV might explain the superantigen-like stimulation of RCS cells was examined. Northern blots of RNA extracted from primary RCS, various RCS tissue-culture lines (cRCS), normal and LPS-stimulated LN B cells were hybridized with MMTV-LTR or ENV probes derived from the C3H exogenous MMTV. A prominent 1.8-kb band was detected in transplantable as well as primary RCS (Fig. 4A). Normal or LPS-activated B cells from SJL mice did not show this mRNA but exhibited small amounts of two larger mRNAs (4.1 kb and 2.9 kb), the smaller of which was increased upon LPS stimulation, similar to that described for

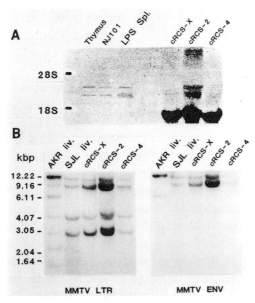

FIGURE 4 Hybridization patterns of MMTV-LTR and -ENV. (A) Northern blot of RNA, extracted from SJL thymus, NJ101, LPS-activated SJL splenic B cells (LPS Spl.), and in vitro RCS lines (cRCS-X, -2, and -4), probed with MMTV-LTR. (B) Southern blot of *Pvu*II-digested genomic DNA extracted from AKR liver, SJL liver, and cRCS lines (cRCS-X, -2, and -4), probed with MMTV-LTR or MMTV-ENV. Size markers (1-kb ladder) are indicated on the left.

normal B cells in other strains (King and Corley 1990; King et al. 1990; Lund and Corley 1991). RCS cells also contained a larger transcript of approximately 9 kb, which was similar to that described for MMTV transcripts in endotoxin-stimulated CH12 B-cell tumors (King and Corley 1990; King et al. 1990; Lund and Corley 1991) and in the MMT mammary tumor cell line (Lund and Corley 1991).

Southern blots of *Eco*RI-, *Pvu*II-, *Bgl*II-, and *Kpn*I-digested genomic DNA from SJL liver, primary RCS, and cRCS lines were probed with C3H MMTV-LTR or ENV. The DNA from primary RCS and from one of the cloned cRCS lines (cRCS-4) did not show any rearranged bands as compared to liver DNA, although all three of these lymphomas had high expression of the 1.8-kb mRNA. DNA from cRCS-2 and cRCS-X, both long-transplanted lymphomas, showed one or two additional bands, dissimilar from each other. Of the four bands hybridizing with MMTV-LTR in liver and RCS-4 DNA digested with *Eco*RI, the 5.3-kb and 6.3-kb bands also hybridized with MMTV-ENV, whereas of the four bands of DNA digested with *Kpn*I hybridizing with the LTR probe, the two larger bands hybridized with the ENV probe (not shown). *Pvu*II-digested RCS and liver DNA gave similar hybridization patterns with MMTV-LTR as published for SJL liver DNA (Frankel et al. 1991), of which the larger two bands hybridized with the ENV probe (Fig. 4B).

Mtv-8 has been localized to chromosome 6 (Dyson et al. 1991). However, the chromosomal location of RCS-*Mtv* has not yet been determined. From the MMTV-LTR hybridization pattern of genomic DNA, it is clear that there are only two endogenous *Mtv*s present in SJL mice (*Mtv-8* and RCS-*Mtv*). SJL mice have been tentatively typed to have *Mtv-29* in their genome (Frankel et al. 1991), but definite proof that this SJL *Mtv* is *Mtv-29* awaits nucleotide sequencing of *Mtv-29* from another strain, such as AKR. The findings in Figure 4B show that although AKR liver DNA digested with *Pvu*II shows two non-*Mtv-8* bands of similar size as SJL liver DNA hybridizing with MMTV-LTR, the larger one of the two hybridizes with MMTV-ENV in the SJL pattern and not in the AKR pattern. It thus seems unlikely that the RCS-*Mtv* is identical to one of the AKR *Mtv*s.

The recently derived Ia[+] B-cell lymphoma, NJ101, which arose in an aged anti-CD4-treated SJL mouse (Lin et al. 1992), exhibits very different properties from RCS: It expresses surface IgM and, in contrast to RCS (Carswell et al. 1976; Ponzio et al. 1986), it grows at least as well in γ-irradiated as in normal SJL mice (V.K. Tsiagbe and G.J. Thorbecke, unpubl.). NJ101 was therefore established in vitro, where it grew without the aid of added γ-irradiated syngeneic T cells, in contrast to cRCS (Lasky et al. 1988). RNA from this in vitro line was examined for the presence of MMTV transcripts. Like normal B cells, it exhibited the 4.1-kb and 2.9-kb mRNA, but not the 1.8-kb transcript seen in RCS. Thus, the ability of the Ia[+] B-cell lymphomas to stimulate T cells (Fig. 1A) correlates with the expression of the 1.8-kb mRNA for MMTV (Fig. 4A).

CHARACTERIZATION OF RCS-Mtv LTR

A cDNA library prepared from cRCS-2 was probed with MMTV-LTR and MMTV-ENV. Three positive clones were amplified and sequenced. When the sequence of the RCS-*Mtv* LTR was compared with that of *Mtv-8* LTR, the usual high degree of homology seen among different *Mtv* genes (Brandt-Carlson et al. 1993; Tsiagbe et al. 1993b) was noted, as was a lack of homology in the 3′ polymorphic region of the open reading frame.

To determine whether the abnormally expressed 1.8-kb mRNA in RCS cells was of *Mtv-8* or of RCS-*Mtv* origin, synthetic oligonucleotides were prepared according to the 3′ polymorphic regions of *Mtv-8* (30-mer), *Mtv-6* (30-mer), and RCS-*Mtv* (31-mer). These were used to probe Northern blots of RNA from normal SJL LN and from cRCS-4. The *Mtv-8*-specific probe hybridized with the 4.1-kb and 2.9-kb mRNA in both normal LN and RCS, whereas the RCS-*Mtv*-specific probe only hybridized with the 1.8-kb mRNA in cRCS-4, a different RCS line from the one used to prepare the cDNA library. The *Mtv-6*-specific probe failed to hybridize with any of the bands (negative control, Tsiagbe et al. 1993b).

For comparison, the predicted amino acid sequence of the carboxy-terminal region of RCS-*Mtv* ORF is shown in Table 2, lined up with a few different *Mtv* ORFs, each representative of a group with similar carboxyl termini. The carboxy-terminal sequence of RCS-*Mtv* ORF extends beyond the others in length (total ORF length 325 amino acids), and it differs significantly from all the others. The most homologous one appears to be *Mtv-7*, which is in the same group as the LTR ORF from SW-21-*Mtv*. Brandt-Carlson et al. (1993) show the multiple alignment of a large number of *Mtv*s in the absence of the sequence of RCS-*Mtv*, suggesting that a gap is needed in all the other ORF sequences to allow for the tryptophan in the *Mtv-7* sequence group at position 311. However, on aligning with RCS-*Mtv* LTR, a gap in the *Mtv-8*, C3Hx-*Mtv*, and DBA/2-*Mtv-6* of 3 amino acids is inserted by the GAP program of GCG, whereas *Mtv-7* has two homologies with RCS-*Mtv* in this region (positions 308 and 310). In this new alignment we have now eliminated the gap at position 311, because a number of new homologies show up when aligned in this way.

TABLE 2 COMPARISON OF PREDICTED CARBOXY-TERMINAL AMINO ACID SEQUENCE OF RCS-MTV LTR-ORF WITH THOSE OF OTHER MTVS

Mtv-ORF	Amino acid position				Vβ specificity
	290 →	300 →	310 →	320 →	
RCS-Mtv	NFWGKFFDYTEEGAIAKILHNKKHTFADKLGMDKLHFT				16
Mtv-7	.....I.........Y.M.Y.HGGRV.F.PF				6, 7, 8.1, 9
C3H-Mtv-8	.V...I.H..K...V.RQ.E---.IS..TF..SYNG				11
C3Hx-Mtv	HF...I.H-.K..TV.GLIE---.YS.KTY..SYYE				14, 15
DBA/2-Mtv-6	-IHW.V.YNSR.E.KRH.IE---.IK.LP.AF				3, 5.1, 5.2

Derived from Tsiagbe et al. (1993b). Representative amino acid sequences of carboxy-terminal polymorphic regions that confer TCR Vβ specificity, from four groups of MMTVs, are shown for comparison with RCS-Mtv. Dashed lines were inserted within some of the sequences in the polymorphic regions to maximize the sequence alignments. Dots indicate there is no amino acid replacement compared to RCS-Mtv. The amino acid sequences of the other Mtvs were derived from published sequences (Mtv-7, Beutner et al. 1992; C3H-Mtv-8, Donehower et al. 1983, C3Hx-Mtv and DBA/2-Mtv-6, Pullen et al. 1992; corrected sequence compilation of MMTVs, Brandt-Carlson et al. 1993). The TCR Vβ specificity information was derived from Beutner et al. (1992) (Vβ6, -7, -8.1, and -9); Dyson et al. (1991) (Vβ11); Choi et al. (1991) (Vβ14 and -15); Woodland et al. (1991) (Vβ3, -5); Gollob and Palmer (1992) (Vβ3, -5.1, and -5.2).

ROLE OF RCS-SPECIFIC MMTV-LTR ORF PRODUCTS IN SYNGENEIC T-CELL STIMULATION

To ascertain the biological significance of this MMTV-LTR expression, the effect of antisense oligonucleotides on syngeneic T-cell-stimulating ability of RCS cells was examined. The homology in the 5′ regions of all *Mtv* LTR sequences so far examined is very high (Held et al. 1992) and, in particular, the sequences around the two most 5′ ATG sites are identical for all *Mtvs* including RCS-*Mtv* and *Mtv-8* (King et al. 1990; Gollob and Palmer 1992; Tsiagbe et al. 1993b). Oligonucleotides, prepared according to the sequences of the two most 5′ potential translation initiation sites, hybridized to the 1.8-kb RNA in RCS lymphomas (not shown), suggesting that antisense oligonucleotides to these regions might interact with the MMTV-LTR transcripts that are present in RCS (Tsiagbe et al. 1993b).

RCS-X cells were first γ-irradiated and then incubated overnight (18–24 hr) with 0.2–1.0 μM antisense or sense S-oligonucleotides. They were then used as stimulator cells in a mixed lymphocyte response with normal SJL LN cells (Fig. 5). As compared to the sense S-oligomers, the antisense S-oligomers, BF1 and BF2, caused a significantly greater inhibition of the ability of cRCS-X to stimulate T cells. A stronger inhibition was observed with the antisense BF2 than with antisense BF1. Addition of antisense BF1 or BF2 to responder LN cells did not affect their responses to Con-A or to 0.025% glutaraldehyde-fixed RCS cells (not shown). In this way, a direct effect of the S-oligomers on the responder cells was excluded.

The availability of the I-A^s-bearing NJ101 cell line, which neither expressed the RCS-specific MMTV-LTR nor was able to stimulate SJL T cells, provided a perfect host cell for transfection experiments with the cloned cDNA for RCS-MMTV. Indeed, after transient transfection with plasmid pSG5 containing the RCS-MMTV-LTR under the β-globin promoter, NJ101 cells were strongly stimulatory for the Vβ16$^+$ RCS-specific T-cell hybridoma, 1D1-E7, whereas NJ101 cells transfected with the empty plasmid were not stimulatory (Fig. 1B) (Tsiagbe et al. 1993b).

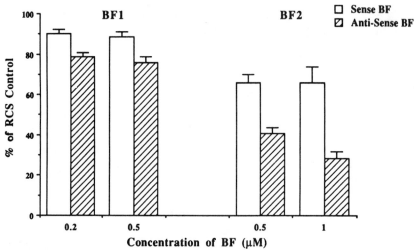

FIGURE 5 Inhibition of RCS stimulation of syngeneic T cell ($[^3H]$TdR incorporation) by two 19-mer antisense S-oligonucleotides prepared according to the sequences of the first (BF1) and second (BF2) translation initiation sites common to RCS-*Mtv* and *Mtv-8*. cRCS-X (7000 rads, 10^4 cells/well) were cultured with oligonucleotides in serum-free AIM V medium, for 24 hr after which 2×10^5 normal LN cells were added to the wells, and cultures were continued for another 90 hr. Control cultures received the equivalent sense S-oligonucleotide. The results were expressed as percentage of responses to RCS not pretreated with BF.

ROLE OF MMTV-LTR ORF AS AN ONCOGENE IN SJL LYMPHOMAS

These results show that RCS cells transcribe an MMTV-LTR ORF which is different from and additional to that transcribed under normal conditions in SJL lymphoid cells, and that this mRNA codes for a superantigen involved in the stimulation of Vβ16+CD4+ T cells by RCS cells. In view of the inhibitory effect of anti-I-A^s, the putative ORF product of the 1.8-kb mRNA seen in RCS cells is likely to stimulate syngeneic Vβ16 cells in association with I-A^s. In I-E+ F_1 hybrid mice, Vβ16+ T cells are largely deleted (Vacchio and Hodes 1989), thus accounting for the absence of responding T cells and of RCS growth in such F_1 hybrids (Ponzio et al. 1986). It should be realized, however, that I-E alone is not effective at causing deletion of Vβ16+ T cells, since I-E transgenic SJL mice do not delete Vβ16 T cells

(Fig. 3B), in line with their ability to support RCS growth (Tsiagbe et al. 1991). These findings demonstrate a novel oncogenic role for endogenous MMTV, mediated by the product of the LTR ORF and its stimulatory properties for Vβ16[+] T cells, since without the cytokine products of the stimulated T cells, SJL lymphomas do not grow (Fig. 6).

Our results are in conflict with those of Katz et al. (1988), who have reported the detection of I-E-like antigen on RCS cells (Ohnishi and Bonavida 1986) and Vβ17a T cells as the major RCS-responsive T-cell subset. This aspect has been discussed at greater length elsewhere in our publications, demonstrating that I-E is absent from RCS (Brown et al. 1983; Brown and Thorbecke 1985) and that Vβ17a T cells are not important in the response to the RCS cell lines studied in our laboratory (Tsiagbe et al. 1991, 1993a). In view of the identification of MMTV-LTR ORF as a superantigen on RCS for Vβ16 T cells, it is unlikely that RCS lines in different laboratories have different properties in this respect.

The mechanism whereby RCS cells start expressing this ORF product needs further study. It is not clear whether this expression also occurs in a small subset of normal SJL B cells, such as, for instance, germinal center cells, from which RCS are thought to arise (Siegler and Rich 1968; Pattengale and

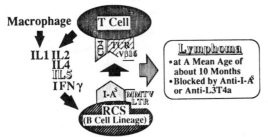

FIGURE 6 Schematic representation of the reversed immunological surveillance essential for growth of SJL follicular center B-cell lymphomas. RCS lymphomas expressing an RCS-*Mtv* LTR ORF product together with I-A[s] stimulate CD4[+], Vβ16[+] syngeneic T cells, which in turn respond by producing cytokines on which the lymphomas depend for growth: All in vitro RCS lines respond to IL-5, some also to IL-4 or IL-2. IL-1 (probably macrophage-derived) is needed for optimal cytokine responses, and IFN-γ synergizes with IL-5 (Lasky and Thorbecke 1989).

Taylor 1983; Tsiagbe et al. 1992), or is peculiar to RCS cells and thus the result of some other gene activation occurring during the lymphomagenesis in SJL mice.

The sequence of the cloned cDNA for RCS-*Mtv* in the 3' regulatory region does not show any deletions or overt differences from other MMTVs. In fact, the three glucocorticoid response elements (TGTTCT) in positions 1035–1040, 1112–1117, and 1127–1132 are identical to those in the *Mtv-8* sequence (King et al. 1990). Thus, although we cannot exclude point mutation(s), enhanced transcription is not likely to be caused by the same mechanism as that responsible for the high transcription of MMTV(GR) in T-cell lymphomas of GR mice, where a large deletion starting in the 3' end of the coding region and extending into the untranslated region is responsible for the enhanced transcription (Theunissen et al. 1989). Translocation of the RCS-*Mtv* is also unlikely as a cause, since there is lack of rearrangements in the MMTV-LTR hybridization patterns of *Eco*RI-, *Bgl*II-, *Kpn*I-, or *Pvu*II-digested genomic DNA from primary RCS and from the recently derived cloned in vitro line, cRCS-4, although they do express the enhanced mRNA for RCS-*Mtv*. Rearrangements of DNA encoding MMTV sequences were seen in two of the long-transplanted RCS lines, which also show a few chromosomal abnormalities (Sopchak et al. 1989; V.K. Tsiagbe et al., unpubl.). Thus, DNA rearrangement of MMTV coding regions is probably not the cause of the enhanced transcription of RCS-*Mtv* in SJL lymphomas. It is also unlikely that infection with an exogenous MMTV could have played a role, since no additional DNA hybridizing with LTR or ENV probes was detected in RCS-4 as compared to liver DNA.

The response to normal Mls-antigen-bearing B cells is relatively self-limiting, in that it is followed by anergy of the responding cells (Speiser et al. 1990; Webb and Sprent 1990; Blackman et al. 1991), whereas the response to RCS cells growing in SJL mice appears to continue and to be needed for the sustained RCS growth (Ponzio et al. 1986). This may be related to the observations that RCS cells are excellent APC (Tsiagbe et al. 1993a). Thus, the costimulatory properties of RCS cells may differ from those of normal splenic B cells, rendering them more apt to activate T cells in a cytokine-productive manner, thereby avoiding the induction of anergy (Schwartz 1990; Liu et al. 1992). In preliminary studies (J. Asakawa and G.J. Thorbecke, unpubl.), we have found that neonatal injection of γ-irradiated RCS cells fails to induce detectable unresponsiveness to RCS. In addition, in previous studies we found only a transient decrease in splenic proliferative responses after repeated intravenous injections of γ-irradiated RCS in adult mice (Ponzio et al. 1977b). Preliminary studies on the presence of costimulatory molecules on the surface of RCS as compared to normal and LPS-activated B cells suggest that, indeed, B7 expression on RCS cells is high. In addition, the initial exposure to RCS may cause a differentiation of the Vβ16+ T cells to memory Th2-type cells. Such cells may be more resistant to the induction of anergy and/or apoptosis and may continue to produce IL-5 and IL-4 on stimulation, as has been suggested previously (Gilbert et al. 1990; Williams et al. 1990). Primary RCS, although they ultimately kill the host, generally are slow-growing and indolent in their behavior. In vivo regression can be obtained by treatment with anti-CD4 (Ohnishi and Bonavida 1987; Alisauskas and Ponzio 1989), suggesting a continued requirement for responding CD4 T cells for lymphoma growth. Therefore, it is possible that the response to RCS is primarily maintained by newly formed thymic Vβ16+ migrants and/or by Th2 memory cells, but that some of the peripheral Vβ16+ T cells indeed do become anergic or apoptotic after contact with RCS.

ACKNOWLEDGMENTS

We are indebted to Drs. P. Marrack and J.W. Kappler (National Jewish Center of Immunology, Denver, Colorado) for anti-Vβ2 (B20.6), anti-Vβ3 (KJ25), anti-Vβ17a (KJ23a); for the KLH-specific, I-A^s-restricted T hybridoma (SK23-7.4); and for the alloreactive T hybridoma (3D0-54.8). We also thank Drs. D. Mathis and C. Benoist (Faculte de Medecine, Strassbourg Cedex, France) for generously providing Eα16 transgenic mice; Dr. O. Kanagawa (Washington University School of Medicine, St. Louis, Missouri) for anti-Vβ6 (RR4-7); Dr. I.E. Weissman (Stanford University School of Medicine, Stanford, California) for anti-Vβ7 (TR310); Dr. D.H. Raulet (Massachusetts Institute of Technology, Cambridge, Massachusetts) for anti-Vβ14 (14-4); Dr. E. Palmer (National Jewish Center of Immunology, Denver, Colorado) for DNA probes: Vβ1, -4, -10, -15, -16, -17, and Cβ, for Vβ16$^+$ T hybridomas, and for anti-Vα2 antibody. Dr. N. M. Ponzio (Department of Pathology, University of Medicine and Dentistry, New Jersey Medical School, Newark, New Jersey) kindly donated the NJ101 lymphoma line for these experiments. These studies were supported by the National Cancer Institute (grants CA-14462, CA-22247, and CA-31346), and the National Institute of Diabetes, Digestive, and Kidney Diseases, U.S. Public Health Service. S.Y.C. was the recipient of a summer fellowship from the American Academy of Allergy and Immunology. Computing was supported by the National Science Foundation under grant DIR-8908095.

REFERENCES

Acha-Orbea, H., A.N. Shakhov, L. Scarpellino, E. Kolb, V. Muller, A. Vessaz-Shaw, R. Fuchs, K. Blochlinger, P. Rollini, J. Billotte, M. Sarafidou, H.R. MacDonald, and H. Diggelmann. 1991. Clonal deletion of Vβ14-bearing T cells in mice transgenic for mammary tumour virus. *Nature* **350:** 207.

Alisauskas, R.M. and N.M. Ponzio. 1989. T-helper-cell-specific monoclonal antibody inhibits growth of B-cell lymphomas in syngeneic SJL/J mice. *Cell. Immunol.* **119:** 286.

Beutner, U., W.N. Frankel, M.S. Cote, J.M. Coffin, and B.T. Huber. 1992. Mls-1 is encoded by the long terminal repeat open reading frame of the mouse mammary tumor provirus Mtv-7. *Proc. Natl. Acad. Sci.* **89:** 5432.

Blackman, M.A., T.H. Finkel, J. Kappler, J. Cambier, and P. Marrack. 1991. Altered antigen receptor signaling in anergic T cells from self-tolerant T-cell receptor β-chain transgenic mice. *Proc. Natl. Acad. Sci.* **88:** 6682.

Brandt-Carlson, C., J.S. Butel, and D. Wheeler. 1993. Phylogenetic and structural analyses of MMTV LTR ORF sequences of exogenous and endogenous origins. *Virology* **193:** 171.

Brown, P.H. and G.J. Thorbecke. 1985. Characterization of the molecules on SJL/J lymphomas which stimulate syngeneic T cells. *J. Immunol.* **135:** 3572.

Brown, P.H., D. Mathis, R.E. Cone, P.P. Jones, N.M. Ponzio, and G.J. Thorbecke. 1983. Properties of reticulum cell sarcomas in SJL/J mice. VIII. Prominent role of RCS cell I-A antigens in the stimulation of syngeneic T cells. *Immunogenetics* **18:** 399.

Carswell, E.A., S.P. Lerman, and G.J. Thorbecke. 1976. Properties of reticulum cell sarcomas in SJL/J mice. II. Fate of labeled tumor cells in normal and irradiated syngeneic mice. *Cell. Immunol.* **23:** 39.

Choi, Y., J.W. Kappler, and P. Marrack. 1991. A superantigen encoded in the open reading frame of the 3′ long terminal repeat of mouse mammary tumour virus. *Nature* **350:** 203.

Cooper, H.M., G. Corradin, and Y. Paterson. 1988. The heme moiety of cytochrome c is an autoreactive Ir gene-restricted T cell epitope. *J. Exp. Med.* **168:** 1127.

Donehower, L.A., B. Fleurdelys, and G.L. Hager. 1983. Further evidence for the protein coding potential of the mouse mammary tumor virus long terminal repeat: Nucleotide sequence of an endogenous proviral long terminal repeat. *J. Virology* **45:** 941.

Dyson, P.J., A.M. Knight, S. Fairchild, E. Simpson, and K. Tomonari. 1991. Genes encoding ligands for deletion of Vβ11 T cells cosegregate with mammary tumour virus genomes. *Nature* **349:** 531.

Frankel, W., C. Rudy, J.M. Coffin, and B.T. Huber. 1991. Linkage of Mls genes to endogenous mammary tumour viruses of inbred mice. *Nature* **349:** 526.

Gilbert, K.M., K.D. Hoang, and W.O. Weigle. 1990. Th1 and Th2 clones differ in their response to a tolerogenic signal. *J. Immunol.* **144:** 2063.

Gollob, K.J. and E. Palmer. 1992. Divergent viral superantigens delete Vβ5[+] T lymphocytes. *Proc. Natl. Acad. Sci.* **89:** 5138.

Hayama, T., N.M. Ponzio, C. Nagler, J. Vilcek, R.F. Coico, and G.J. Thorbecke. 1984. Ia-restricted interaction of normal lymphoid cells and SJL lymphoma (reticulum cell sarcoma) leading to lymphokine production. III. Relative roles of reticulum cell sarcoma and normal lymphoid cells in lymphokine production. *J. Natl. Cancer Inst.* **72:** 321.

Held, W., A.N. Shakhov, G. Waanders, L. Scarpellino, R. Luethy, J.-P. Kraehenbuhl, H.R. MacDonald, and H. Acha-Orbea. 1992. An exogenous mouse mammary tumor virus with properties of Mls-1 (Mtv-7). *J. Exp. Med.* **175:** 1623.

Katz, I.R., J. Chapman-Alexander, E.B. Jacobson, S.P. Lerman, and G.J. Thorbecke. 1981. Growth of SJL/J-derived transplantable reticulum cell sarcoma as related to its ability to induce T-cell proliferation in the host. III. Studies on thymectomized and congenitally athymic SJL mice. *Cell. Immunol.* **65:** 84.

Katz, I.R., S.P. Lerman, N.M. Ponzio, D.C. Shreffler, and G.J. Thorbecke. 1980. Growth of SJL/J-derived transplantable reticulum cell sarcoma as related to its ability to induce T-cell proliferation in the host. I. Dominant negative genetic influences of other parent haplotype in F_1 hybrids of SJL/J mice. *J. Exp. Med.* **151:** 347.

Katz, J.D., K. Ohnishi, L.T. Lebow, and B. Bonavida. 1988. The SJL/J T cell response to both spontaneous and transplantable syngeneic reticulum cell sarcoma is mediated predominantly by the $V\beta17a^+$ T cell clonotype. *J. Exp. Med.* **168:** 1553.

King, L.B. and R.B. Corley. 1990. Lipopolysaccharide and dexamethasone induce mouse mammary tumor proviral gene expression and differentiation in B lymphocytes through distinct regulatory pathways. *Mol. Cell. Biol.* **10:** 4211.

King, L.B., F.E. Lund, D.A. White, S. Sharma, and R.B. Corley. 1990. Molecular events in B lymphocyte differentiation. Inducible expression of the endogenous mouse mammary tumor proviral gene, Mtv-9. *J. Immunol.* **144:** 3218.

Kozak C., G. Peters, R. Pauley, V. Morris, R. Michalides, J. Dudley, M. Green, M. Davisson, O. Prakash, A. Vaidya, J. Hilgers, A. Verstraeten, N. Hynes, H. Diggelmann, D. Peterson, J.C. Cohen, C. Dickson, N. Sarkar, R. Nusse, H. Varmus, and R. Callahan. 1987. A standardized nomenclature for endogenous mouse mammary tumor viruses. *J. Virol.* **61:** 1651.

Lamont, A.G., A. Sette, R. Fujinami, S.M. Colon, C. Miles, and H.M. Grey. 1990. Inhibition of experimental autoimmune encephalomyelitis induction in SJL/J mice by using a peptide with high affinity for IA^s molecules. *J. Immunol.* **145:** 1687.

Lasky, J.L. and G.J. Thorbecke. 1989. Characterization and growth factor requirements of SJL lymphomas. II. Interleukin 5 dependence of the in vitro cell line, cRCS-X, and influence of other cytokines. *Eur. J. Immunol.* **19:** 365.

Lasky, J.L., N.M. Ponzio, and G.J. Thorbecke. 1988. Characterization and growth factor requirements of SJL lymphomas. I. Development of a B cell growth factor-dependent in vitro cell line, cRCS-X. *J. Immunol.* **14:** 679.

Lerman, S.P., E.A. Carswell, J. Chapman, and G.J. Thorbecke. 1976. Properties of reticulum cell sarcomas in SJL/J mice. III. Promotion of tumor growth in irradiated mice by normal lymphoid cells. *Cell. Immunol.* **23:** 53.

Lerman, S.P., J. Chapman-Alexander, D. Umetsu, and G.J. Thorbecke. 1979. Properties of reticulum cell sarcomas in SJL/J mice. VII. Nature of normal lymphoid cells proliferating in response to tumor cells. *Cell. Immunol.* **43:** 209.

Lin, T-Z., H. Fernandes, R. Yauch, N.M. Ponzio, and E. Raveche. 1992. IL-10 production in a $CD5^+$ B cell lymphoma arising in a CD4 monoclonal antibody treated SJL mouse. *Clin. Immunol. Immunopathol.* **65:** 10.

Liu, Y., B. Jones, A. Aruffo, K.M. Sullivan, P.S. Linsley, and C.A. Janeway, Jr. 1992. Heat-stable antigen is a costimulatory molecule for CD4 T cell growth. *J. Exp. Med.* **175:** 437.

Lopez, D.M., V. Charyulu, and R.D. Paul. 1985. Regulated expression of mouse mammary tumor proviral genes in cells of the B lineage.

J. Immunol. **134:** 603.

Lund, F.E. and R.B. Corley. 1991. Regulated expression of mouse mammary tumor proviral genes in cells of the B lineage. *J. Exp. Med.* **174:** 1439.

Molina, I.J., N.A. Cannon, R. Hyman, and B.T. Huber. 1989. Macrophages and T cells do not express Mls determinants. *J. Immunol.* **143:** 39.

Ohnishi, K. and B. Bonavida. 1986. Mapping of SJL/J reticulum cell sarcoma tumor-associated Ia antigens by T cell hybridomas: Characterization of tumor-specific and shared epitopes detected on IE⁺ allogeneic cells. *J. Immunol.* **137:** 733.

———. 1987. Regulation of Ia⁺ reticulum cell sarcoma (RCS) growth in syngeneic SJL/J mice. I. Inhibition of tumor growth by passive administration of L3T4 monoclonal antibody before or after tumor inoculation. *J. Immunol.* **138:** 4524.

Pattengale, P.K. and O.R. Taylor. 1983. Experimental models of lymphoproliferative disease. The mouse as a model for human non-Hodgkin's lymphomas and related leukemias. *Am. J. Pathol.* **113:** 237.

Ponzio, N.M., A. Alonso, and R.M. Alisauskas. 1987. Dependence of lymphoma growth on "reversed immunological surveillance". *Pathol. Immunopathol. Res.* **6:**1.

Ponzio, N.M., P.H. Brown, and G.J. Thorbecke. 1986. Host-tumor interactions in the SJL lymphoma model. *Int. Rev. Immunol.* **1:** 273.

Ponzio, N.M., J. Chapman-Alexander, and G.J. Thorbecke. 1978. Properties of reticulum cell sarcomas in SJL/J mice. VI. Characterization of lymphoid cells that proliferate in response to RCS cells. *Cell. Immunol.* **41:** 157.

Ponzio, N.M., C.S. David, D.C. Shreffler, and G.J. Thorbecke. 1977a. Properties of reticulum cell sarcomas in SJL/J mice. V. Nature of reticulum cell sarcoma surface antigen which induces proliferation of normal SJL/J T cells. *J. Exp. Med.* **146:** 132.

Ponzio, N.M., S.P. Lerman, J.M. Chapman, and G.J. Thorbecke. 1977b. Properties of reticulum cell sarcomas in SJL/J mice. IV. Minimal development of cytotoxic cells despite marked proliferation to syngeneic RCS *in vivo* and *in vitro. Cell. Immunol.* **32:** 10.

Ponzio, N.M., T. Hayama, C. Nagler, I.R. Katz, M.K. Hoffmann, K. Gilbert, J. Vilcek, and G.J. Thorbecke. 1984. Ia-restricted interaction of normal lymphoid cells and SJL lymphoma (reticulum cell sarcoma) leading to lymphokine production. II. Rapid production of antibody-enhancing factor, interleukin 2, and immune interferon. *J. Natl. Cancer Inst.* **72:** 311.

Pullen, A.M., Y. Choi, E. Kushnir, J. Kappler, and P. Marrack. 1992. The open reading frames in the 3′ long terminal repeats of several mouse mammary tumor virus integrants encode Vβ3-specific superantigens. *J. Exp. Med.* **175:** 41.

Schwartz, R.H. 1990. A cell culture model for T lymphocyte clonal anergy. *Science* **248:** 1349.

Shimonkevitz, R., J. Kappler, P. Marrack, and H. Grey. 1983. Antigen recognition by H-2-restricted T cells. I. Cell-free antigen processing. *J. Exp. Med.* **158:** 303.

Siegler, R. and M.A. Rich. 1968. Pathogenesis of reticulum cell sarcoma in mice. *J. Natl. Cancer Inst.* **41:** 125.

Sopchak, L., S.R. King, D.A. Miller, N. Gabra, G.R. Thrush, and S.P. Lerman. 1989. Progression of transplanted SJL/J lymphomas attributed to a single aggressive H-2D-negative lymphoma. *Cancer Res.* **49:** 665.

Speiser, D., E.Y. Chvatchko, R.M. Zinkernagel, and H.R. MacDonald. 1990. Distinct fates of self-specific T cells developing in irradiation bone marrow chimeras: Clonal deletion, clonal anergy, or *in vitro* responsiveness to self-Mls-1^a controlled by hemopoietic cells in the thymus. *J. Exp. Med.* **172:** 1305.

Stavnezer, J.L. Lasky, N.M. Ponzio, M.P. Scheid, and G.J. Thorbecke. 1989. Reticulum cell sarcomas of SJL mice have rearranged immunoglobulin heavy and light chain genes. *Eur. J. Immunol.* **19:** 1063.

Tax, A., D. Ewert, and L.A. Mason. 1983. An antigen cross-reactive with gp52 of mammary tumor virus is expressed on a B cell subpopulation of mice. *J. Immunol.* **130:** 2368.

Theunissen, H.J.M., M. Paardekooper, J. Maduro, R.J.A. Michalides, and R. Nusse. 1989. Phorbol ester-inducible T-cell-specific expression of variant mouse mammary tumor virus long terminal repeats. *J. Virol.* **63:** 3466.

Tsiagbe, V.K. and G.J. Thorbecke. 1990. Paraproteins and primary lymphoma in SJL mice. I. Individuality of idiotypes on paraproteins. *Cell. Immunol.* **129:** 494.

Tsiagbe, V.K., J. Asakawa, and G.J. Thorbecke. 1993a. The syngeneic response to SJL follicular center B cell lymphoma (RCS) cells is primarily in Vβ16$^+$, CD4$^+$ T cells. *J. Immunol.* **150:** 5519.

Tsiagbe, V.K., J.L. Rabinowitz, and G.J. Thorbecke. 1991. I-E Expression does not by itself influence growth of or T cell unresponsiveness to SJL lymphomas. *Cell. Immunol.* **136:** 329.

Tsiagbe, V.K., M. Nicknam, H.D. Fattah, and G.J. Thorbecke. 1992. IL-5 responsive subsets among normal and lymphomatous murine B cells. *Ann. N.Y. Acad.Sci.* **651:** 270.

Tsiagbe, V.K., T. Yoshimoto, J. Asakawa, S.Y. Cho, D. Meruelo, and G.J. Thorbecke. 1993b. Linkage of superantigen-like stimulation of syngeneic T cells in a mouse model of follicular B cell lymphoma to transcription of endogenous mammary tumor virus. *EMBO J.* **12:** 2313.

Vacchio, M.S. and R.J. Hodes. 1989. Selective decreases in T cell receptor Vβ expression. Decreased expression of specific V families is associated with expression of multiple MHC and non-MHC gene products. *J. Exp. Med.* **170:** 1335.

Webb, S.R. and J. Sprent. 1990. Induction of neonatal tolerance to Mls^a antigens by CD8$^+$ T cells. *Science* **248:** 1643.

Williams, M.E., A.H. Lichtman, and A.K. Abbas. 1990. Anti-CD3 antibody induces unresponsiveness to IL-2 in Th1 clones but not in Th2 clones. *J. Immunol.* **144:** 1208.

Woodland, D.L., M.P. Happ, K.J. Gollob, and E. Palmer. 1991. An endogenous retrovirus mediating deletion of αβ T cells? *Nature* **349:** 529.

Superantigenicity of Rabies Virus Nucleocapsid in Humans and Mice

M. Lafon,[1] **D. Scott-Algara,**[2] **E. Jouvin-Marche,**[3]
and P.N. Marche[3]

[1]Unité de la Rage, [2]Unité d'Immunohématologie
et d'Immunopathologie, [3]Unité d'Immunochimie analytique
CNRS UA 359, Institut Pasteur, 75724 Paris cedex 15, France

Both endogenous and exogenous mouse mammary tumor viruses (Mtvs and MMTVs) were found to exhibit superantigen properties (Acha-Orbea and Palmer 1991; Huber 1992; Acha-Orbea et al. 1993). The open reading frame (ORF) in the 3′ long terminal repeat (LTR) of the mouse Mtvs encodes self-superantigens that induce clonal deletion of T lymphocytes (Acha-Orchea et al. 1991; Choi et al. 1991; Woodland et al. 1991). The translation product corresponds to a type II transmembrane glycoprotein (Korman et al. 1992). No viral superantigen has been identified so far in humans, although superantigen-like properties have been suggested for human immunodeficiency virus 1 (HIV-1) (Janeway 1991). We have recently shown that the nucleocapsid (NC) of the rabies virus induces specific Vβ8 human T lymphocyte proliferation and binds to HLA class II molecules (Lafon et al. 1992). We had also previously established that the NC was a potent activator for human peripheral blood lymphocytes (PBL) (Herzog et al. 1992). Taken together, these data provide evidence that the NC of the rabies virus is an exogenous virus superantigen in humans. Rabies virus can infect all mammals, and rabies virus strains have been adapted to laboratory mice. Therefore, we investigated whether rabies NC was also a superantigen in mice. Preliminary results of NC-induced deletion and clonal expansion of Vβ T cells indicate that NC is indeed a superantigen in mice. Mice appear to be a suitable model in which to further characterize NC properties. This model will be help-

Superantigens: A Pathogen's View of the Immune System
© 1993 Cold Spring Harbor Laboratory Press 0-87969-398-3/93 $5 + .00

ful to investigate in particular the NC capacity to stimulate an immune response and the role it could play in rabies virus pathogenicity.

PHYSICAL PROPERTIES OF NC AND N PROTEIN

Rabies virus, a bullet-shaped rhabdovirus (Fig. 1A), contains a single negative-strand RNA molecule that codes for five proteins, the N, NS, G, M, and L proteins. G and M are envelope proteins. Only G protein is exposed on the surface of the virion and forms spikes protruding through the virus envelope. The three internal proteins, N, NS, and L, together with the viral RNA, constitute the NC (Fig. 1C). The NC forms a 165-nm x 50-nm helical structure with 30–35 coils in virions (Murphy 1975) and can measure up to 4.6 µm when liberated after breakage of the virus envelope (Fig. 1A, B) (Sokol et al. 1969). N protein is estimated to be 54 kD–62 kD by SDS-PAGE. Slight discrepancies with the predicted molecular weight deduced from the 450-amino-acid length are probably due to the effect of phosphate groups attached to serine residues (Dietzschold et al. 1987a). Despite the existence of potential N-glycosylation sites, N protein is not glycosylated (Dietzschold 1977). N protein, tightly associated with the rabies virion RNA genome, protects the RNA from ribonucleases and ensures a suitable configuration for transcription (Wunner 1991). In the present study, both NC and its major constituent, the N protein, were tested for superantigen properties. NC was purified from rabies-virus-infected-hamster (BSR) cell lysates through CsCl gradients as described previously (Lafon and Wiktor 1985). The N protein was produced in insect cells (*Spodoptera frugiperda*, Sf9) infected with a baculovirus expression vector containing the complete coding region of the N-protein gene of the rabies virus (Préhaud et al. 1990). Infected cell lysates were purified through a 5–20% glycerol gradient as described previously (Préhaud et al. 1990).

Superantigenic properties of recombinant N protein were contained in the heaviest fractions of glycerol gradients. Electron microscopy analysis indicated these fractions contain rosettes of 8–12 molecules; no RNA was found associated with

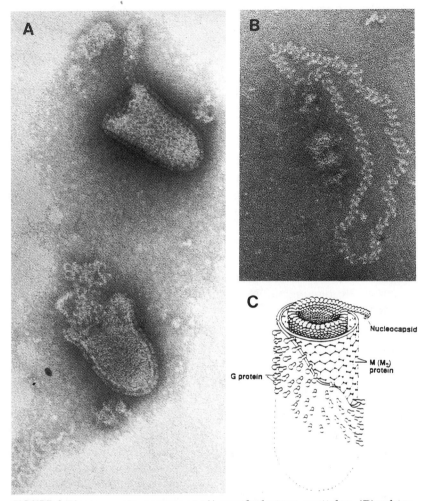

FIGURE 1 Electron microscopy of (A) purified virus particles, (B) rabies NC purified by CsCl from rabies-infected hamster fibroblasts (magnification, 200,000x). (C) schematic diagram of rabies virus showing the envelope of virus surrounding the NC structure. In panel A, the top virus particle is intact, whereas the lower particle is liberating NC.

these structures (C. Préhaud, per. comm.). Extracts of mock-infected cells treated by the same purification procedure did not support T-cell proliferation. Cell cultures and virus seed lots were mycoplasma-free. Taken together, these data rule out the possibility that cellular contaminants could be responsible for the rabies virus superantigen property.

BINDING OF NC AND N PROTEIN TO THE HUMAN MHC CLASS II MOLECULES

Binding of NC and N-protein to MHC class II αβ complexes expressed on the surface of different cell lines was analyzed by flow cytometry (Fig. 2). Mouse fibroblasts (NIH-3T3) expressing human major histocompatibility complex (MHC) class II αβ DR molecules (Korman et al. 1987) and control cells were incubated at 4°C for 60 minutes successively with 10 μg of N protein or NC, anti-N protein monoclonal antibody (MAb) and fluorescein isothiocyanate (FITC) F(ab′)₂ goat anti-mouse IgG. As shown in Figure 2, N protein binds to the surface of mouse fibroblasts expressing MHC class II molecules but not to nontransfected fibroblasts, indicating that N protein does bind to

FIGURE 2 (*A,B*) MHC class II molecule expression is required for cell-surface NC binding and N protein binding. NC and N protein binding was determined by surface immunofluorescence (*A*) on human DR-transfected mouse fibroblasts and (*B*) on the human MHC class-II-negative 721 x CEM-T2 cell line (Salter et al. 1985), the class-II-positive B-cell line 309, the DP⁺ cell line 721-84-5 (DeMars 1984), and the DQ⁺ cell line CL-13 mutants (Ono et al. 1991). Cells (2 x 10⁶) were incubated at 4°C for 60 min, with 10 μg of NC or N protein, anti-N-protein MAb (PVA3) (Lafon and Wiktor 1985), and FITC F(ab′)₂ goat anti-mouse IgG. Binding was analyzed in EPICS flow cytometer as follows: Results are presented as mean (M) and peak (Pk) of fluorescence for each profile obtained after incubation with NC or N protein (solid lines). Percentages of positive cells were obtained after subtraction of negative controls—without NC or N-protein incubation (dashed lines). The mean and the peak in negative controls were, respectively: 38,14 (panel *1*); 42,11 (panel 2); 61,64 (panel 3); 50,63 (panel 4); 33,12 (panel 5); 29,14 (panel 6); 47,13 (panel 7); and 50,63 (panel 8). HLA phenotypes of the 309 cell line are DR13/7, DQ1/2. For the 721-84-5 cell line, phenotypes are DP2/- and CL-13 DQ1/1. (Reprinted, with permission, from Lafon et al. 1992 [copyright Macmillan Magazines Ltd.].) (*C*) Class-II-negative Raji B-cell line exhibits additional superantigen receptors. N protein binding was determined by surface immunofluorescence on the human MHC class-II-positive Raji cell line and its MHC class-II-negative variant, RJ2.5.2. As shown in the top panel, these two types of cells exhibit differential surface MHC class II expression, whereas N protein binding was not abolished in the MHC class II mutant (bottom panel). Both parental and variant Raji cell lines expressed a high level of surface IgG (data not shown).

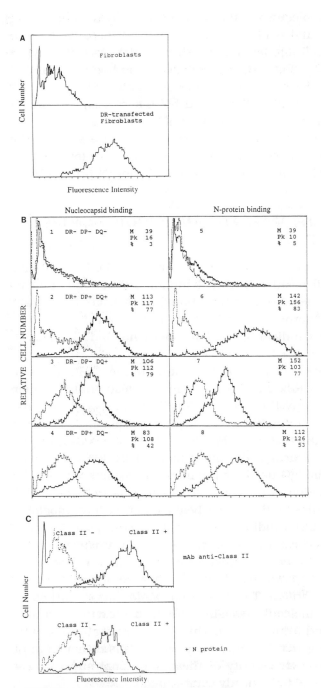

FIGURE 2 (*See facing page for legend.*)

MHC class II molecules. This was confirmed by the absence of binding of NC and N protein with a class-II-negative human T x B hybrid cell line lacking the three major class II isotypes (DR⁻, DP⁻, DQ⁻) (Fig. 2B, top panels). In addition, NC and N protein bind to B-cell variants expressing either HLA DQ or DP isotypes only (Fig. 2B, middle and bottom panels). NC and N protein also bind to the cell surface of several B-cell lines with different HLA types (data not shown). These data support the assumption that there is no absolute requirement for a particular MHC class II allele or isotype for NC and N protein binding.

ADDITIONAL RECEPTORS FOR NC AND N PROTEIN ON THE SURFACE OF B CELLS

Binding of NC and N protein on the surface of the Raji cell line, a MHC class-II-positive Burkitt lymphoma B-cell line, and its MHC class-II-negative variant RJ2.2.5 (Accola 1983) was tested in cytofluorometry. In contrast to the previous observation (Fig. 2A,B) indicating that NC does not bind a class-II-negative human T x B hybrid cell line lacking the three major class II isotypes, N protein did bind to the MHC class-II-negative variant RJ2.2.5 (Fig. 2C). This suggests that N protein recognizes not only the major MHC class II isotypes, but also other cell-surface molecules present on Epstein-Barr virus (EBV)-immortalized B cells (Fig. 2C). Moreover, in blotting experiments, NC reacts with components of 92 kD and 69 kD identified as the IgG used for the immunoprecipitation of class II molecules (Lafon et al. 1992). This suggests that these cell-surface molecules could be the heavy chain of immunoglobulins (Fraser 1992). Binding of bacterial superantigen to similar high-molecular-weight components, so-called "unspecific binding," has been reported previously (see, e.g., Mollick et al. 1989). It is noteworthy that another superantigen, the *Mycoplasma arthritidis* T-cell mitogen, MAM, has a marked affinity for high-molecular-weight molecules present in culture media (Cole and Atkins 1991). This should indicate that binding to IgG is a general feature of superantigens rather than an exception. However, identity of these additional superantigen receptors remains to be firmly established.

IN VITRO SELECTIVE EXPANSION OF HUMAN Vβ8 T CELLS IN HUMANS

To study the specificity of NC and N protein for human T-cell receptors (TCR) with particular Vβs, PBL from unprimed and rabies-primed individuals were analyzed for Vβ expression after various in vitro stimulations (Table 1). PBL of unprimed donors (Table 1a) and of rabies-vaccinated donors (primed donors) (Table 1b) were stimulated with N protein or NC, or not stimulated. Cells were stained with anti-Vβ MAbs and analyzed by flow cytometry. For each individual, N protein and NC significantly increased the percentage of T cells bearing Vβ8, whereas T cells bearing other Vβs were unchanged. No preferential Vβ patterns were observed when PBL from rabies-vaccinated donors were stimulated with entire inactivated virus particles or phytohemagglutinin (PHA), suggesting that the virus particles, in contrast to NC, do not engage T cells that bear particular TCR Vβs. The importance of Vβ8 T cells in the NC-specific response was analyzed by studying the remaining reactivity of Vβ8-depleted PBL populations. The Vβ8-positive T cells were removed from the PBL by using the anti-Vβ8-specific MAb coupled to magnetic beads. Vβ usage and proliferation were measured in Vβ8-depleted PBL, enriched-Vβ8 T cells, and nondepleted PBL cultivated with virus particles or NC (Fig. 3). Nondepleted and Vβ8-depleted PBL responded to the virus. The decreased proliferative response of the depleted population correlates with the absence of Vβ8 T cells (Fig. 3A). The NC induced a powerful proliferation response of PBL, which was abolished by the depletion of Vβ8 lymphocytes (Fig. 3B). The lack of proliferation of the Vβ8-depleted PBL indicates that Vβ8-negative T-cell subpopulations do not respond to NC under these conditions.

Vβ8-enriched T cells (attached to the beads) were cultured in the presence of virus particles or NC without addition of antigen-presenting cells (APCs). Proliferation was only observed after NC stimulation, showing that, unlike virus particles, processing is not required for the presentation of NC to T cells. A double signal provided by anti-Vβ8 MAb and NC could stimulate the T cells through an unconventional pathway previously suggested for microbial toxin superantigen (Liu et al.

TABLE 1 SELECTIVE EXPANSION OF Vβ8 T CELLS AFTER IN VITRO NC OR N PROTEIN STIMULATION

(a) Unprimed donors

	Donor 1		Donor 2			Donor 3			Donor 4			Donor 5			Donor 6		
	-N	+N	-N	+N	+NC	-N	+N	+NC	-N	+N	+NC	-N	+N	+NC	-N	+N	+NC
Vβ5a	3.2	4.3	2.4	2.2	2.2	3.1	3.3	3.1	3.2	2.5	2.7	2.3	2.6	3.0	2.3	2.4	2.9
Vβ5b	-	-	-	-	-	-	-	-	-	-	-	1.1	0.8	1.3	1.2	0.8	0.9
Vβ6,-7	4.1	4.2	2.6	2.1	2.3	1.7	1.7	1.8	1.9	1.6	1.4	4.5	3.6	3.6	0.4	0.6	0.7
Vβ8	3.6	8.4	2.2	5.6	5.5	2.4	6.2	5.8	3.1	6.5	6.1	4.5	9.1	9.0	1.8	3.2	4
Vβ12	5.7	4.9	2.2	2.3	2.3	1.3	1.5	1.2	2.8	3.5	0.9	5.2	4.2	4.6	1.6	1.5	1.5

(b) Rabies-primed donors

	Donor 1			Donor 2			Donor 3			Donor 4			Donor 5			Donor 6	
	V	PHA	NC	V	PHA	NC	V	PHA	NC	V	PHA	NC	V	PHA	NC	-N	+N
Vβ5	2.4	2.2	2.0	0.8	0.7	0.6	2.2	3.0	3.4	2.6	2.4	1.1	2.4	2.6	1.6	4.7	4.3
Vβ5b	0.7	0.9	1.0	-	-	-	1.9	2.0	2.4	1.9	2.0	1.4	-	-	-	-	-
Vβ6,-7	2.3	2.3	1.9	2.0	2.8	1.6	2.3	2.7	2.7	3.2	2.5	1.6	2.0	2.3	2.0	2.3	3.1
Vβ8	3.4	4.0	9.4	3.4	3.2	7.0	5.0	5.6	10.2	4.8	5.3	11.4	3.2	2.8	4.9	4.	8.2
Vβ12	2.4	2.7	1.1	4.0	3.9	2.4	0.8	1.4	1.0	2.8	3.5	0.9	1.2	1.0	0.7	5.1	4.8

Vβ usage in PBL from 6 unprimed donors (a) and 6 primed (rabies-vaccinated) donors (b) was estimated by cytofluorometry before stimulation (-N) or after stimulation (day 9) with 5 μg/ml recombinant N protein, NC, rabies virus particles (V), or with PHA. Recombinant IL-2 (5 units/ml) was added on day 4 and day 8. Cells (2 x 10^6) were incubated at 4°C with anti-Vβ MAbs or anti-TCR MAb and FITC-(Fab')$_2$ anti-mouse IgG and analyzed with an EPICS-752 flow cytometer gated to exclude nonviable cells. Usage of a given Vβ was expressed as percentage of TCR-positive T cells determined with the anti-TCR MAb WT31. Anti-Vβ MAbs were from T-Cell Sciences (anti-Vβ5a: 1C1; anti-Vβ5b: W112; anti-Vβ6: OT145; anti-Vβ8: 16G8; and anti-Vβ12: S511). Irrelevant IgGs were used as negative controls. (Reprinted, with permission, from Lafon et al. 1992.)

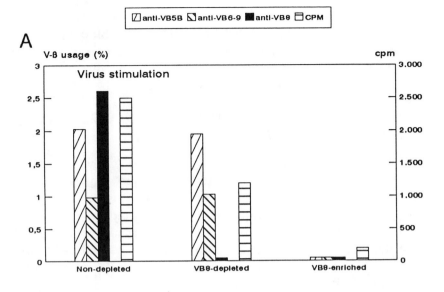

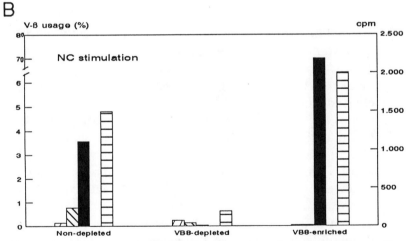

FIGURE 3 Depletion of Vβ8 T lymphocytes abolishes NC-specific proliferation. PBL were incubated with anti-Vβ8 MAb, then with Dynabeads coated with sheep anti-mouse IgG antibodies. Cells attached to the beads were isolated with a magnet. Nondepleted PBL, Vβ8-depleted PBL, and Vβ8-positive T cells were maintained in culture with virus (*A*) or NC (*B*) without addition of APCs. Recombinant IL-2 was added on day 4. Staining with anti-Vβ5b, -6–9, and -8 MAbs was performed on day 10. Proliferation assays, performed as described previously (Herzog et al. 1992), were measured on day 8. (Reprinted, with permission, from Lafon et al. 1992 [copyright Macmillan Magazines Ltd.].)

1991). However, activated human T cells can express MHC class II molecules essential for superantigen binding and subsequent T-cell proliferation. The purification procedure and culture conditions may induce MHC class II expression on Vβ8 T cells, which could then function as APCs.

IN VIVO SELECTIVE EXPANSION OF Vβ6 AND Vβ7 T CELLS IN ADULT BALB/c MICE

To analyze the specificity of NC for mouse TCR with particular Vβs, we used the local injection technique, which leads to a very strong local immune response in the draining lymph node (Held et al. 1992). Adult BALB/c 7-week-old mice, free of exogenous MMTVs, were injected in the footpad with 50 μg of NC diluted in medium (RPMI-1640), or medium alone. After injection (3, 5, and 10 days) popliteal lymph nodes were removed, and percentages of lymph node cells (LNCs) bearing Vβ6, -7, -10, or -14 TCR were estimated by cytofluorometry. After NC inoculation (3 days), the draining popliteal lymph nodes increased in size about fivefold in comparison with lymph nodes of naive mice. The percentages of Vβ6, -7, -10, and -14 T cells were estimated among blasts and resting T cells. As shown in Figure 4, the percentage of CD4$^+$ blasts expressing Vβ6 increased from 12.8 ± 1.7% in control (day 0) to 23.4 ± 0.9% at day 3. In some experiments, NC injection led to an increase of Vβ6 reaching up to 60% of the CD4$^+$ blasts. Similarly, percentages of blasts expressing Vβ7 increased from 4.65 ± 0.25% up to 12.5 ± 0.6% at day 3. After a peak response at day 3, percentages of T cells bearing Vβ6 and Vβ7 declined and returned to normal levels 10 days after injection. In contrast, percentages of blasts expressing Vβ14 or Vβ10 remained unchanged throughout the course of the experiment (Fig. 4). Percentages of T cells bearing Vβ6 and Vβ7 among the LNCs of small and intermediate size (resting T cells) were not modified (data not shown), indicating that the Vβ T-cell increase results from a specific activation process.

NEONATAL DELETION IN BALB/c MICE

During the maturation of T cells in the thymus, T cells that interact strongly with self-MHC molecules are eliminated by a

% CD4 V beta usage

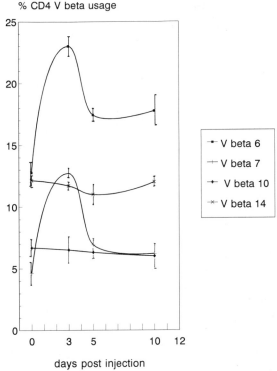

days post injection

FIGURE 4 Kinetic analysis of Vβ6, -7, -10, and -14 usage by CD4+ popliteal LNCs. LNCs were harvested from naive and NC-injected adult BALB/c mice, teased, and incubated with one of the following biotinylated MAbs (anti-Vβ6, -7, -10, and -14) (Acha-Orbea et al. 1993). FITC-conjugated antibody to CD4 (MAb GK1.5) was used as a second step in conjunction with phycoerythrin (PE)-conjugated strep-tavidin. LCNs were analyzed in a FACScan cytofluorimeter (Becton-Dickinson) (Jouvin-Marche et al. 1992). Blast CD4+ T cells were gated by forward and side-scatter analysis. Values given are the results of means of four different animals in two separate experiments ± S.E.M. For control (day 0), LNCs of three naive animals were pooled.

process called "negative selection." In mice expressing Mls antigen, the Mls-reactive T cells are deleted by negative selection due to self-cross-reactivity (Kappler et al. 1988; MacDonald et al. 1988). Injection of bacterial superantigen into neonatal mice leads to the deletion of the reactive mature T cells in the thymus (White et al. 1989). Deletion of self-reactive cells can also be observed in the periphery (Jones et al. 1990, Webb et al. 1990).

To study the clonal deletion induced by the rabies super-antigen, BALB/c mice were injected intraperitoneally every other 2 days after birth during 2 weeks with 50 µg of purified NC. Mothers were systematically tested for the absence of known exogenous MMTVs. Percentages of Vβ2–11, -14, and -17 T cells from thymus and spleen from both normal and NC-injected animals were estimated by cytofluorometry 4 and 8 weeks after birth. Mature thymocytes were enriched by treatment of mice 2 days before sacrifice with injection of hydrocortisone. Hydrocortisone has been shown to increase the effect of superantigen-mediated neonatal deletion by decreasing the cytokine release necessary to support superantigen-driven stimulation (Lussow et al. 1993). As shown in Figure 5A, 8 weeks after birth, in the NC-injected animals, percentages of CD3$^+$ thymocytes expressing Vβ2, -6, -7, -8.3, and -14 decreased by twofold in comparison to percentages in their normal littermates. In spleens (Fig. 5B), Vβ6, -7, -8.3, and -14 CD4$^+$ T cells showed a 50% decrease 4 weeks after birth. Peripheral deletion of Vβ2 was not studied in this experiment.

Our results show that NC engages in mice a selective expansion of at least Vβ6 and -7 and a deletion of Vβ2, -6, -7, -8.3, and -14 T cells. Although our data are incomplete since Vβ2 and Vβ8 local expansion has not been studied, it is noteworthy that there is already a slight discrepancy between

FIGURE 5 Neonatal deletion in BALB/c mice injected with NC. Analysis of TCR usage by CD3$^+$ thymocytes (*A*) and CD4$^+$ splenocytes (*B*) of NC-inoculated mice (black bars) and of their normal littermates (white bars). Baby mice were inoculated intraperitoneally every other day after birth with 50 µl of RPMI-1640 medium containing 50 µg of NC, or with medium alone. Both normal and NC-inoculated mice were injected intraperitoneally with 1 mg of hydrocortisone 2 days before analysis. Splenocytes and thymocytes from both medium- and NC-injected animals were double-stained with one of the following biotinylated Vβ-specific MAbs (Vβ2–11, -14, and -17) (Marrack and Kappler 1990; Acha-Orbea et al. 1993) and in a second step with PE-conjugated-streptavidin and FITC-conjugated anti-CD4 or anti-CD3 MAbs. Cells were analyzed in a FACScan flow cytometer. Values given correspond to a single control and a single NC-injected animal.

the results of Vβ expansion and those of deletion. Indeed, CD3$^+$ Vβ14 and CD4$^+$ Vβ14 are partially deleted in thymus and spleen, respectively (Fig. 3), whereas the level of CD4$^+$ Vβ14 remains unchanged in lymph nodes (Fig. 4). One poten-

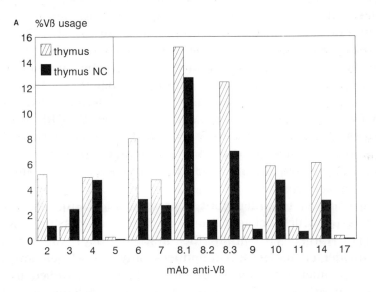

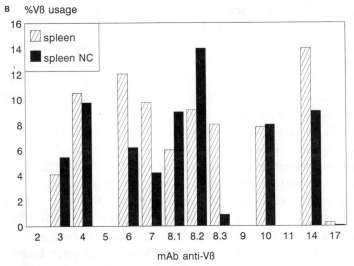

FIGURE 5 (*See facing page for legend.*)

tial explanation is that Vβ14 T cells are deleted not because Vβ14 T cells are rabies superantigen targets, but because NC reactivates a silent integrated MMTV. Each laboratory mouse strain and most wild-derived mouse strains have integrated MMTV genomes. Among the 43 Mtvs that have been identified so far (Kozak et al. 1987), some of them, such as Mtv-1 or Mtv-2, retained the capacity of inducing infectious virus particles and mammary tumors (Dickson 1985). At this point, it cannot be ruled out that the BALB/c mice we used bore a not-yet-described integrated mouse retrovirus encoding a Vβ14-specific superantigen, which NC reactivates by an unknown mechanism. In contrast, the alternative hypothesis that the BALB/c mice we used were infected by maternally inherited MMTV transmitted by milk, such as MMTV (GR), which deletes Vβ14, can be clearly excluded because normal littermates exhibited normal Vβ14 percentages in both thymus and spleens (6% among CD3$^+$ thymocytes and 12% among CD4$^+$ splenocytes).

In contrast to endogenous expressed superantigens, such as Mls-1a, which delete virtually all T cells expressing superantigen target Vβ within the first 10 days after birth (Schneider et al. 1989), NC induces only partial deletion. In the experiments we reported, Vβ deletion was studied in 1- and 2-month-old BALB/c mice. At this age, deletion of Vβ14 was not achieved either in MMTV(GR) transgenic or in chronically infected mice (Acha-Orbea et al. 1991; Ignatowicz et al. 1992). In these mice, superantigen deletion settled gradually and was never complete. The partial deletion of Vβ6 and Vβ11 T cells, reported in some strains of mice, was presented as evidence of Vα TCR involvement in superantigen recognition (Tomonari and Fairchild 1991; Vacchio et al. 1992).

Similarly, the partial deletion induced by rabies NC may result in a weak interaction of NC with TCR, indicating that additional variable components of the TCR including Vα are required. Another possible explanation is that NC does not penetrate well into the thymus cortex and does not affect cells with moderate affinity. However, it cannot be excluded that some potential NC-reactive T cells had time to escape deletion because they matured in the first 2 days after birth before the superantigen injections had started.

CONCLUSIONS AND FUTURE DIRECTIONS

Our results clearly establish that rabies NC triggers a preferential stimulation of Vβ T cells both in humans after in vitro activation (Vβ8) and in vivo in mice after local injection (Vβ6, Vβ7). Moreover, in baby mice, repeated injections of NC lead to the peripheral elimination of the particular Vβs (Vβ6 and Vβ7) preferentially stimulated by NC. Since NC binds to surface class II molecules and does not require processing (Lafon et al. 1992), the results obtained in the mouse model strengthen our conclusion that rabies NC is a superantigen. However, a number of important issues remain to be solved: (1) Why do phylogenetically unrelated microorganisms, like rabies, *M. arthritidis*, and MMTV, stimulate and delete the same Vβs? (2) Why does rabies virus encode a superantigen? and (3) Can rabies NC superantigen be involved in the immunostimulatory properties of NC described previously (Dietzschold et al. 1987b)?

1. In mice expressing Mls-1a, bearing integrated Mtv-7 or Mtv-43 genomes, or in mice infected with MMTV-SW, the majority of Vβ6, -7, -8-1, and -9 T cells are deleted from the mature CD4+ thymocytes as well as from peripheral T cells (MacDonald et al. 1988; Acha-Orbea et al. 1991). *M. arthritidis* mitogen MAM preferentially stimulates Vβ6 and Vβ8. Our finding that NC also targeted Vβ6, -7, and -8 addresses the question why phylogenetically unrelated microorganisms stimulate and delete the same Vβs. It has not been shown yet that the same site of Vβ6 interacts with the three superantigens. If this is the case, the origin of this functional similarity should be investigated. Functional similarity in the absence of sequence homologies has been exemplified with enterotoxins SE and TSST-1 (Marrack and Kappler 1990). It has been speculated that the secondary structure of a protein may enhance its attachment to the cell-surface receptor. Thus, despite low structural homologies between SE toxins and TSST-1, it has been postulated that a similar pattern of secondary structures (low α-helix and high β-sheet content) may explain their common reactivities (Johnson et al. 1991). It remains to be established whether similar secondary structures in ORF,

MAM, and NC sequences may explain their common reactivity.

2. In vivo superantigen stimulation is known to induce widespread proliferation followed by an immunosuppression as a consequence of anergy and peripheral deletion in superantigen-reactive T cells and, possibly, as a consequence of massive release of cytokines. It has been postulated that MMTV could utilize superantigen properties to paralyze the host immune system and enhance the viral invasion (Acha-Orbea and Palmer 1991; Palmer 1991). One possibility is that the host cannot control the virus invasion because of the immune paralysis induced by the virus-encoded superantigen. Alternatively, viral superantigen can stimulate Vβ T cells, which are natural targets of the virus.

Rabies virus evades the host immune response because of its intrinsic neurotropism and its capacity to induce a very minor host reaction. The weakness of the primary immune response could be the result of poor virus replication at the site of inoculation. It could also be the result of the virus capacity to immunosuppress the host defenses. T lymphocytes play an important role in immune defense against rabies. Demonstration that rabies virus is a T-dependent antigen was established by experiments in T-lymphocyte-deficient athymic (nude), immunosuppressed, and lymphocyte-reconstituted mice (Turner 1976; Smith 1981). We address the question of whether the presence of NC superantigen is a hallmark of the capacity of rabies virus to weaken the local immune reaction.

Because rabies NC specifically stimulates Vβ8 human T cells, we recently investigated the possibility that Vβ8 human T cells are specific targets for rabies virus infection. Rabies virus can infect the human Jurkat lymphoblastoid T-cell line expressing Vβ8 TCR, but also T-cell lines missing TCR. This indicates that Vβ8 T cells are not a preferential lymphoblastoid target of rabies virus infection (J. Montano-Hirose and M. Lafon, pers. comm.). If rabies superantigen plays any role in rabies-associated immunosuppression, it is not documented yet. In contrast, previous studies on mouse resistance to rabies virus infection showed that mouse strains display differences in susceptibility to rabies.

Lodmel (1983) demonstrated that SJL (H-2^s) or CBA (H-2^k) mice were highly resistant to infection by a rabies virus, whereas C57BL/6 (H-2^b), ASW (H-2^s), or A/WY (H-2^a) were highly susceptible. It cannot be excluded that Ir genes play a role in this resistance. However, it is intriguing to note that the genetically resistant mice delete several Vβs, including Vβ6, -7, -9, and -11, whereas susceptible mice like C57BL/6 do not. One can hypothesize that in resistant strains of mice, superantigen-mediated immune paralysis could not be effective because of the absence of relevant Vβ T cells. In contrast, in susceptible mice, superantigen could efficiently turn off the host immune system because of the presence of adequate Vβ T cells.

3. Superantigen-like properties of rabies virus NC and N protein could have considerable effects on vaccinal strategy. NC and N protein of rabies virus, like other internal antigens (influenza, measles), can protect animals and enhance the production of neutralizing antibodies directed to the viral envelope proteins (Scherle and Gerhard 1986; Dietzschold et al. 1987b; Bankamp et al. 1991; Herzog et al. 1992).

This property raises the question of how rabies NC can be a protective molecule and a superantigen simultaneously. Generally speaking, enterotoxin superantigens have a negative effect on antibody production. Thus, in vivo SEB decreases both T- and B-cell responses (Pinto et al. 1978), and in vitro SEB inhibits antibody production by the human IgA-secreting B-cell line MOPC-315. However, at low concentrations, SEB suppresses both rat and mouse proliferative responses to mitogen; at high concentrations (10–50 μg/ml), it strongly stimulates the mouse T-lymphocyte proliferative response (Ben-Nun and Yossefi 1992), indicating that doses are important in the nature of superantigen effects. Moreover, mediated B-cell activation was also reported. In particular, superantigens, like MAM and TSST-1, did not exhibit any suppressive effect in vivo on B-cell functions; rather, they activated resting B cells in vitro, induced polyclonal B-cell proliferation and immunoglobulin secretion (Mourad et al. 1989; Tumang et al. 1990), and, in vivo, increased the number of antibody-producing cells in response to the injection of sheep red blood cells (Cole and Atkins 1991). Therefore, for the rabies NC, the association of suppressant and stimulatory properties might not be so paradoxical. Protection conferred by rabies NC could reflect the expansion of CD4$^+$ Vβ6, Vβ7 T lymphocytes involved in the production of virus-neutralizing antibodies. It would be assumed in that case that, contrary to bacterial superantigens, rabies NC can induce cognate T-B interactions leading to enhancement of the immune response. However, since clonal expansion of T cells could be followed by anergy, further in vivo studies are necessary to characterize the effects of NC super-antigenicity on vaccinal strategy.

ACKNOWLEDGMENTS

Mireille Lafage and Danielle Voegtlé are acknowledged for expert technical assistance. We thank Andres Alcover for the Raji cell line and its negative MHC class II mutant, Charly Dauguet for electronic microscopy, Alan Korman for the human MHC class-II-transfected mouse fibroblast cell line, Gérard Orth for critically reviewing the manuscript, and Christophe Préhaud for communication of unpublished results. E.J.-M. and P.N.M. are investigators from INSERM.

REFERENCES

Accola, R.S. 1983. Human B cell variants immunoselected against a single Ia antigen subset have lost expression of several Ia antigen subsets. *J. Exp. Med.* **157:** 1053.

Acha-Orbea, H. and E. Palmer. 1991. Mls-A retrovirus exploits the immune system. *Immunol. Today* **12:** 356.

Acha-Orbea, H., W. Held, G.A. Waanders, A.N. Shakhov, L. Scarpellino, R.K. Lees, and H.R. MacDonald. 1993. Exogenous and endogenous mouse mammary tumor virus superantigens. *Immunol. Rev.* **131:** 5.

Acha-Orbea, H., A.N. Shakhov, L. Scarpellino, E. Kolb, V. Müller, A. Vessaz-Shaw, K. Blöchinger, P. Rollini, J. Billote, M. Sarafidou, H.R. MacDonald, and H. Diggelmann. 1991. Clonal deletion of

Vβ14 positive T cells in mammary tumor virus transgenic mice. *Nature* **350**: 207.

Bankamp, B., U.G. Brinckmann, A. Reich, S. Niewiesk, V. ter Meulen, and U.G. Liebert. 1991. Measles virus NC protein protects rats from encephalitis. *J. Virol.* **65**: 1695.

Ben-Nun, A. and S. Yossefi. 1992. Staphylococcal enterotoxin B as a potent suppressant of T lymphocytes: Trace levels suppress T lymphocytes proliferative responses. *Eur. J. Immunol.* **22**: 1495.

Choi, Y., J.W. Kappler, and P. Marrack. 1991. A superantigen encoded in the open reading frame of the 3′long terminal repeat of mouse mammary tumor virus. *Nature* **350**: 203.

Cole, B.C. and C.L. Atkins. 1991. The *Mycoplasma arthritidis* T cell mitogen, MAM: A model superantigen. *Immunol. Today* **12**: 271.

DeMars, R. 1984. Mutations that dissect the D-region of a human B lymphoblastoid cell line. *Dis. Markers* **2**: 175.

Dickson, C. 1985. Molecular aspects of mouse mammary tumor virus biology. *Int. Rev. Cytol.* **108**: 119.

Dietzschold, B. 1977. Oligosaccharides of the glycosylation of rabies virus. *J. Virol.* **23**: 286.

Dietzschold, B., M. Lafon, H. Wang, L. Otvos, E. Celis, W.H. Wunner, and H. Koprowski. 1987a. Localization and immunological characterization of antigenic domains of the rabies N and NS proteins. *Virus Res.* **8**: 103.

Dietzschold, B. , H. Wang, C.E. Rupprecht, E. Celis, M. Tollis, H. Ertl, E. Heber-Katz, and H. Koprowski. 1987b. Induction of protective immunity against rabies by immunization with rabies virus ribonucleoprotein. *Proc. Natl. Acad. Sci.* **84**: 9165.

Fraser, J. 1992. Superantigen data. *Nature* **360**: 423.

Held, W., A.N. Shakhov, G. Waanders, L. Scarpellino, R. Luethy, J.-P. Kraehenbuhl, H.R. MacDonald, and H. Acha-Orbea. 1992. An exogenous mouse mammary tumor virus with properties of Mls1-a (MTV-7). *J. Exp. Med.* **175**: 1623.

Herzog, M., M. Lafage, J.A. Montano-Hirose, C. Fritzell, D. Scott-Algara, and M. Lafon. 1992. NC specific T and B cell responses in humans after rabies vaccination. *Virus Res.* **24**: 77.

Huber, B.T. 1992. Mls genes and self-superantigens. *Trends Genet.* **8**: 399.

Ignatowicz, L., J. Kappler, and P. Marrack. 1992. The effects of chronic infection with a superantigen-producing virus. *J. Exp. Med.* **175**: 917.

Janeway, C.A. 1991. *Mls*: Makes a little sense. *Nature* **349**: 459.

Johnson, H.M., J.K. Russell, and C.H. Pontzer. 1991. Staphylococcal enterotoxin microbial superantigens. *FASEB J.* **5**: 2706.

Jones, L.A., L.T. Chin, D.L. Longo, and A.M. Kruisbeek. 1990. Peripheral clonal elimination of functional T cells. *Science* **250**: 1726.

Jouvin-Marche, E., P.-A. Cazenave, D. Voegtle, and P.N. Marche.

1992. Vβ17 T-cell deletion by endogenous mammary tumor virus in wild-type derived strains. *Proc. Natl. Acad. Sci.* **89:** 3232.

Kappler, J.W., U.D. Staerz, J. White, and P.C. Marrack. 1988. Self-tolerance eliminates T cells specific for Mls-modified products of the major histocompatibility complex. *Nature* **332:** 35.

Korman, A.J., P. Bourgarel, T. Meo, and G.E Rieckhof. 1992. The mouse mammary tumor virus long terminal repeat encodes a type II transmembrane glycoportein. *EMBO J.* **11:** 1901.

Korman, A.J., J.D. Frantz, J.L. Strominger, and R.C. Mulligan. 1987. Expression of human class II major histocompatibility complex antigens using retrovirus vectors. *Proc. Natl. Acad. Sci.* **84:** 2150.

Kozak, C., G. Peters, R. Pauley, V. Morris, R. Michaelidis, J. Dudley, M. Green, M. Davisson, O. Prakash, A. Vaidya, J. Hilgers, A. Verstaeten, N. Hynes, H. Diggelmann, H. Peterson, J.C. Cohen, C. Dickson, N. Sarkar, R. Nusse, and H. Varmus. 1987. A standardized nomenclature for endogenous mouse mammary tumor viruses. *J. Virol.* **61:** 1651.

Lafon, M. and T.J. Wiktor. 1985. Antigenic structure of the rabies virus NC. *J. Gen. Virol.* **66:** 2125.

Lafon, M., M. Lafage, A. Martinez-Arends, F. Vuillier, V. Lotteau, D. Charron, and D. Scott-Algara. 1992. Evidence in humans of a viral superantigen. *Nature* **358:** 507.

Liu, H., M.A. Lampe, M.V. Iregui, and H. Cantor. 1991. Conventional antigen and superantigen may be coupled to cooperative T cell activation pathways. *Proc. Natl. Acad. Sci.* **88:** 8705.

Lodmel, D. 1983. Genetic control of resistance to street rabies virus in mice. *J. Exp. Med.* **157:** 451.

Lussow, A.R., T. Crompton, O. Karapetian, and H.R. MacDonald. 1993. Peripheral clonal deletion of superantigen-reactive T cells is enhanced by cortisone. *Eur. J. Immunol.* **23:** 578.

MacDonald, H.R., R. Schneider, R.K. Lees, R.C. Howe, H. Acha-Orbea, H. Festenstein, R.M. Zinkernagel, and H. Hengartner. 1988. T-cell receptor Vβ use predicts reactivity and tolerance to Mls1a encoded antigens. *Nature* **332:** 40.

Marrack, P. and J. Kappler. 1990. The staphylococcal enterotoxins and their relatives. *Science* **248:** 705.

Mollick, J.A., R.G Cook, and R.R. Rich. 1989. Class II MHC molecules are specific receptors for staphylococcus enterotoxin A. *Science* **244:** 817.

Mourad, W., P. Scholl, A. Diaz, R. Geha, and T. Chatila. 1989. The staphylococcal toxic shock syndrome toxin 1 triggers B cell proliferation and differentiation via major histocompatibility complex-unrestricted cognate T/B cell interaction. *J. Exp Med.* **170:** 2011.

Murphy, F. 1975. Morphology and morphogenesis of rabies virus. In *The natural history of rabies* (ed. G.M. Baer), vol. 1, p. 33. Academic Press, New York.

Ono, S.J., V. Bazil, M. Sugarawa, and J.L. Strominger. 1991. An isotype-specific trans-acting factor is defective in a mutant B cell line that expresses HLA-DQ but not -DR or -DP. *J. Exp. Med.* **173:** 629.

Palmer, E. 1991. Infectious origins of superantigens. *Curr. Biol.* **1:** 74.

Pinto, M., M. Torten, and S.C. Birnbaum. 1978. Suppression of in vivo humoral and cellular immune response by staphylococcal enterotoxin B. *Transplantation* **25:** 320.

Préhaud, C., R.D. Harris, V. Fulop, C.-L. Koh, J. Wong, A. Flamand, and D.H.L. Bishop. 1990. Expression, characterization and purification of a phosphorylated rabies nucleoprotein synthesized in insect cells by baculovirus vectors. *J. Virol.* **178:** 486.

Salter, R.D., D.N. Howell, and P. Creswell. 1985. Genes regulating HLA class I antigen expression in T-B lymphoblast hybrids. *Immunogenetics* **21:** 235.

Scherle, P.A. and W. Gerhard. 1986. Functional analysis of influenza-specific helper T cell clones in vivo. *J. Exp. Med.* **169:** 1114.

Schneider, R., R.K. Lees, T. Pedrazzini, R.M. Zinkernagel, H. Hengartner, and H.R. MacDonald. 1989. Postnatal disappearance of self reactive (Vβ6$^+$) cells from the thymus of Mls1a mice: Implications for T cell development and autoimmunity. *J. Exp. Med.* **169:** 2149.

Smith, J. 1981. Mouse model for abortive rabies infection of the central nervous system. *Infect. Immun.* **31:** 297.

Sokol, F., H.D. Schlumberger, T.J. Wiktor, H. Koprowski, and K. Hummeler. 1969. Biochemical and biophysical studies on the NC and on the RNA of rabies virus. *Virology* **38:** 651.

Tomonari, K. and S. Fairchild. 1991. The genetic basis of negative selection of Tcrb-V11+ T cells. *Immunogenetics* **33:** 157.

Tumang, J.R., D.N. Posnett, B.C. Cole, M.K. Crow, and S.M. Friedman. 1990. Helper T cell-dependent human B cell differentiation mediated by a mycoplasma superantigen bridge. *J. Exp. Med.* **170:** 2153.

Turner, G.S. 1976. Thymus-dependence of rabies vaccine. *J. Gen. Virol.* **33:** 535.

Vacchio, M.S, O. Kanagawa, K. Tomonari, and R.J. Rhodes. 1992. Influence of T cell receptor Vα expression on Mlsa superantigen-specific T cell responses. *J. Exp. Med.* **175:** 1405.

Woodland, D.L., M.P. Happ, K.J. Gollub, and E. Palmer. 1991. An endogenous retrovirus mediating deletion of $\alpha\beta$ T cells? *Nature* **349:** 529.

Webb, S., C. Morris, and J. Sprent. 1990. Extrathymic tolerance of mature T cells: Clonal elimination as a consequence of immunity. *Cell* **63:** 1249.

White, J., A. Herman, A.M. Pullen, R. Kubo, J.W. Kappler, and P. Marrack. 1989. The Vβ-specific superantigen staphylococcal enterotoxin B: Stimulation of mature T cells and clonal deletion in neonatal mice. *Cell* **56:** 27.

Wunner, W.H. 1991. The chemical composition and molecular structure of rabies viruses. In *The natural history of rabies*, 2nd edition
(ed. G.M. Baer), p. 31. Academic Press, New York.

Superantigens and the Pathogenesis of Viral Diseases

H. Soudeyns,[1] **N. Rebai,**[1] **G.P. Pantaleo,**[2] **F. Denis,**[1] **A.S. Fauci,**[2] **and R.-P. Sékaly**[1]

[1]Laboratoire d'Immunologie, Institut de Recherches Cliniques de Montréal Montréal, Canada, H2W 1R7
[2]Laboratory of Immunoregulation, National Institute of Allergic and Infectious Diseases, National Institutes of Health, Bethesda, Maryland 20892

Superantigens (sAgs) have been recognized on the basis of their inherent capacity to trigger massive activation of an unusually large proportion of CD4$^+$ T cells, stemming from the fact that sAg recognition by T cells operates almost exclusively according to the T-cell receptor (TCR) Vβ chain specificity. Typical T-cell responses to sAgs lack conventional major histocompatibility complex (MHC) restriction, resulting from direct coupling of the sAg to MHC class II molecules at sites different from the polymorphic peptide-binding groove. Presumably, sAgs activate T cells through simultaneous binding of TCR and MHC class II molecules, thereby bridging the T-cell activation complex and triggering the generation of transmembrane signaling pathways associated with T-cell activation.

Molecules that have qualified as sAgs belong in either of two broad groups: Bacterial proteins such as *Staphylococcus aureus* enterotoxins (SEA-SEE, TSST-1) and *Mycoplasma arthritidis* mitogen (MAM) were, respectively, associated with acute toxemias in humans and with infectious arthritis in mice (Marrack and Kappler 1990; Cole and Atkin 1991). Viral gene products (v-sAgs) like the *sag* (3'orf) gene of endogenous and exogenous mouse mammary tumor viruses (MMTV) and the nucleocapsid (N protein) of rabies virus possess genuine superantigenic properties (Choi et al. 1991; Lafon et al. 1992). Several other viruses are now suspected of encoding v-sAgs

(Table 1): EBV, the etiologic agent of infectious mononucleosis, is capable of inducing B-cell and T-cell proliferation in vivo and in vitro (Hanto et al. 1985). HVS encodes a protein with strong sequence homology with the MMTV *sag* gene (Thomson and Nicholas 1991). In vitro superantigenic activity has also been associated with the pr60^{gag} of MAIDS virus (Hügin et al. 1991). Finally, several lines of evidence have suggested that HIV-1, the causative agent of AIDS, could potentially encode a molecule with superantigenic properties (Imberti et al. 1991; Dalgleish et al. 1992; Laurence et al. 1992; Soudeyns et al. 1993).

In many instances, v-sAgs so far described appear instrumental to the pathogenic processes involved in corresponding viral diseases. Thus, v-sAgs represent a new class of pathogenic determinants. In this paper, we attempt to summarize current available knowledge on the involvement of v-sAgs in viral pathogenesis, with emphasis on MMTV and MAIDS virus infections, rabies, and AIDS.

ROLE OF SUPERANTIGENS IN MOUSE MAMMARY TUMORS

Murine minor lymphocyte stimulatory (*Mls*) genes control the generation of mixed lymphocyte reactions between mouse strains that are otherwise fully MHC compatible (Festenstein 1973). This Mls phenotype was attributed to the cell-surface expression of a class of molecules analogous to the MHC, encoded by the *Mls* locus (for review, see Abe and Hodes 1989; Janeway et al. 1989). Recently, these various *Mls* loci were shown to tightly cosegregate with endogenous MMTV proviral integrants (Dyson et al. 1991; Frankel et al. 1991; Woodland et al. 1991). Transfection of class-II-positive cells with constructs comprising the 3' LTR open reading frame (3'orf) of these endogenous MMTVs showed that this gene encodes a protein with superantigenic properties (Choi et al. 1991). The 3'orf gene, renamed *sag* in keeping with the 3-letter nomenclature of retrovirus-derived genes, is also present in exogenous varieties of MMTV (Moore et al. 1987), thereby explaining how exogenous milk-borne MMTVs, like their endogenous relatives, can mediate peripheral Vβ deletions in

TABLE 1 *VIRUSES ENCODING GENUINE OR PUTATIVE v-sAgs*

Virus	Protein	Evidence of v-sAg properties	References
MMTV	sag (3'orf)	genetic linkage with Mls	Marrack et al. (1991); Frankel et al. (1991); Dyson et al. (1991)
		Vβ-specific deletion in vivo	Woodland et al. (1991); Acha-Orbea and Palmer (1991)
		Vβ-specific stimulation in vitro	Choi et al. (1991)
Rabies	nucleocapsid (N protein)	interaction with class II MHC Vβ-specific stimulation in vitro	Lafon et al. (1992)
EBV	unknown	stimulation of T-cell proliferation in vivo	Hanto et al. (1985)
HVS	unknown (early gene?)	sequence homology with MMTV sag	Thomson and Nicholas (1991)
MAIDS	pr60^{gag}	Vβ-specific T-cell proliferation in vitro	Hügin et al. (1991); Kanagawa et al. (1992)
SIV PBJ14	unknown	proliferation of T cells in vivo	Dewhurst et al. (1990); Fultz (1991)
HIV-1	unknown	Vβ repertoire perturbations	Imberti et al. (1991); Dalgleish et al. (1992) Laurence et al. (1992)
		enhanced HIV replication in Vβ12 T cells	

(MMTV) Mouse mammary tumor virus; (EBV) Epstein-Barr virus; (HVS) herpesvirus saimiri; (MAIDS) murine acquired immunodeficiency syndrome; (SIV) simian immunodeficiency virus; (HIV) human immunodeficiency virus.

the progeny of infected female mice (Marrack et al. 1991). *Mls* determinants can associate with MHC class II molecules, although the site of interaction has yet to be identified, and activate T cells on the basis of Vβ-chain specificity alone, via specific interaction with residues of the Vβ chain lying away from conventional complementarity-determining regions (Pullen et al. 1990, 1991).

Until recently, the pathological relevance of the activation-deletion process mediated by MMTV *sag* was unclear. The derivation of mice transgenic for the *sag* gene of exogenous MMTV-C3H (Golovkina et al. 1992) showed that the deletion of Vβ14 T cells consecutive to transgene expression rendered mice immune to superinfection by MMTV-C3H. Therefore, Vβ14 T cells must represent a crucial intermediate target cell for completion of the MMTV life cycle. Since MMTV is known to possess tropism for lymphocytes and a number of other tissue types (Salmons and Gunzburg 1987), it is improbable that replicative restriction takes place at the level of viral entry. More likely, it is the *sag*-mediated Vβ14-specific activation per se that enables MMTV to attain high levels of replication in this specific T-cell subset. The boost in viral replication probably results in enhanced propagation of MMTV to other target tissues, namely mammary epithelium, from which vertical transmission can proceed. Figure 1A depicts the MMTV life cycle.

The nucleotide and amino acid sequence of most MMTV *sag* genes is highly conserved, except in a short carboxy-terminal segment postulated to interact with the TCR. Following infection with MMTV, T cells expressing reactive Vβ determinants are deleted, providing the host with resistance to infection with that particular MMTV. These facts thus suggest that selective pressure has driven the diversification of MMTV v-sAgs, enabling new MMTVs to infect novel T-cell specificities. Conversely, germ-line capture of various MMTV proviruses provides the animal with inherent resistance to a variety of MMTV strains and perhaps significantly limits the diversity of its own peripheral Vβ repertoire. Thus, the MMTV/Mls system appears to be a rare example of equilibrium between a pathogen capable of relatively frequent germ-line access and the immune system of its host, which has the inherent ability to avoid pathogenesis via target cell deletion.

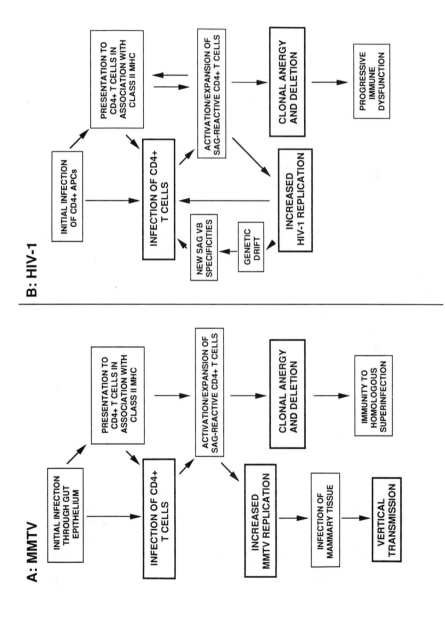

FIGURE 1 Proposed model of pathogenesis induced by MMTV and HIV-1-associated v-sAg.

SUPERANTIGENS IN THE PATHOGENESIS OF MAIDS

MAIDS is characterized by lymphadenopathy, immunosuppression, polyclonal B- and T-cell activation, and aggressive B-cell malignancies, symptoms that are usually associated with AIDS in humans (Mosier et al. 1985; Hügin et al. 1991). MAIDS is caused by a defective type-C oncovirus present in the Duplan isolate of murine leukemia virus (Legrand et al. 1981), which can unexpectedly induce disease in the absence of helper virus (Aziz et al. 1989). MAIDS virus seems to replicate most efficiently in B cells, but it has also been isolated from peripheral CD4$^+$ T cells (Huang et al. 1991; Kubo et al. 1992). The MAIDS virus carries a variant *gag* fusion gene that encodes pr60^{gag}, its specific pathogenic determinant (Huang and Jolicoeur 1990). pr60^{gag}-related polypeptides are found expressed at the surface of B cells and have been shown to confer superantigenic properties specific to T cells expressing TCR Vβ5, -11, and -12 (Hügin et al. 1991; Kanagawa et al. 1992). It is important to keep in mind that all these in vitro experiments were performed on cells infected with both the MAIDS and helper viruses. It is possible that the sAg phenotype could have resulted from indirect effects of other viral functions (i.e., activation of endogenous MMTVs).

Many analogies can be drawn between the life cycle of MAIDS virus and that of MMTV:

1. Both are oncogenic retroviruses that cause tumors in their natural hosts. In fact, tumor production appears instrumental in MAIDS virus-induced pathogenesis, since treatment with cyclophosphamide abrogates disease progression in affected animals (Simard and Jolicoeur 1991).
2. Both viruses can be propagated vertically, and transmission can most efficiently occur via mother's milk (Okada et al. 1992).
3. Both viruses are dependent on specific lymphocyte subsets to generate disease. Indeed, some mouse strains expressing I-E molecules, in which Vβ5, -11, and -12 segments are deleted by endogenous sAgs, are considerably more resistant to MAIDS (Kanagawa et al. 1992).

Since MAIDS virus is grossly defective, it is possible that

homologous recombination events take place with some analogous endogenous murine proviruses, thereby restoring replication competence. This new recombinant retrovirus could potentially encode v-sAg determinants responsible for Vβ-specific target cell deletions. In view of the above-mentioned similarities, it is tempting to postulate that the main purpose of the MAIDS-associated v-sAg is analogous to that served in MMTV, namely, to further viral replication in T-lymphocytic cells, which then act as carriers to spread infection to other pathologically significant target tissues.

SUPERANTIGENS IN RABIES VIRUS INFECTION

Rabies virus belongs to the rhabdoviridae family of minus-strand RNA viruses. It infects an impressive range of mammals, including man, causing acute encephalitis accompanied by severe neuronal degeneration. Rabies virus can infect a variety of cell types, like connective tissue and salivary gland epithelia, but it has a preferred tropism for neural tissue and the central nervous system (CNS) (Baer 1988). In addition, experimental rabies infection in mice is associated with acute lymphocyte depletion, which precedes the appearance of characteristic neurological symptoms, wasting, and death (Torres-Anjel et al. 1988). The use of a murine model has also established that T cells play a role in the neuropathogenesis of animal rabies, since nude mice did not develop paralysis upon rabies virus infection (Sugamata et al. 1992).

In a recent report, sAg activity was attributed to the nucleocapsid protein (N protein) of rabies virus. Using flow cytometric analysis, Lafon et al. (1992) showed that N protein specifically interacted with class-II-positive cells, but not class-II-negative cells. Not only could binding to class-II-positive cells be competed by antibodies directed against MHC class II molecules, but N protein also associated specifically with MHC class II α chains immunoprecipitated with anti-class II monoclonal antibodies. Moreover, purified N protein presented by live or fixed B cells was capable of triggering the selective expansion of Vβ8[+] T cells in vitro. Analogous stimulation upon presentation by fixed B cells suggested that processing of N protein was not required for T-cell proliferation (Lafon et al. 1992). Taken together, these data indicated that rabies virus N protein possessed sAg activity analogous to that of bacterial enterotoxins.

The logic behind the existence of rabies virus-associated sAg activity is not as obvious as in the case of MMTV, which stringently requires a lymphoid host cell intermediate to complete its life cycle. Although severe lymphocytic depletion occurs during the course of rabies induction in susceptible mice, rabies virus is not known to infect lymphocytes to any significant extent. In fact, progression of the virus to the CNS starting from the initial infection site is thought to occur via peripheral ascending axonal travel, a pathway that presumably enables rabies virus to avoid engaging the immune system (Baer 1988). Although hematogenous access of rabies virus to the CNS has been surmised, it has been neither directly demonstrated nor formally disproved. The lymphocytic depletion observed in rabies-infected mice likely resulted from indirect corticosteroid-mediated lymphotoxicity, since proportions of $CD5^+$ and $CD8^+$ cells were unchanged in the infected animal, and adrenalectomy prevented the appearance of this symptom altogether. It is nevertheless intriguing that it is the I-A-bearing lymphocytes (B cells) that were the most significantly affected by the depletion (Perry et al. 1990). It is well known that in sAg-treated mice, sAg-activated cytotoxicity can lead to the killing of bystander cells. Rabies infection of selected mouse strains that have undergone Mls-mediated deletion of the functional equivalents of the human TCR Vβ8 subset could potentially reveal whether this lymphocyte subset is required for efficient disease induction in vivo. Indeed, some mouse strains, like SJL ($H-2^s$), are naturally resistant to experimental infection with rabies virus, and the basis for this lack of susceptibility has not so far been elucidated (Perry et al. 1990; Perry and Lodmell 1991). It is tempting to speculate that the resistance to infection could be due to the large deletion of TCR Vβ-chain genes that is present in SJL mice (Behlke et al. 1986).

Finally, it would be erroneous to assume that replicative advantage and enhanced invasiveness represent the only practical reasons for maintaining a protein with sAg activity. By activating T-cell subsets of mostly irrelevant antigen specificities, rabies virus could conceivably be misguiding the host's immune system, thereby gaining a non-negligible competitive advantage in its race with ongoing immune responses.

SUPERANTIGENS IN HIV-1 INFECTION AND AIDS

Initial infection with HIV-1 is characterized by a transient state of viremia, followed by a latency period of variable duration during which viral replication appears restrained to low levels. During this time, slow progressive depletion of CD4[+] helper-inducer T cells takes place and eventually brings about a profound, unremitting suppression of cell-mediated immunity that is a hallmark of advanced HIV disease and AIDS (Fauci et al. 1984; Fauci 1988). The CD4 molecule specifically binds viral gp120 and acts as the HIV-1 receptor (Klatzmann et al. 1984; Maddon et al. 1986). CD4 is expressed predominantly on T cells, monocytes, oligodendrocytes, and microglial cells in the CNS, although low levels of expression are found in various other cell types (Gartner et al. 1986; Monroe et al. 1988). Several cytopathogenetic mechanisms have been proposed to explain the massive loss of CD4[+] T cells seen in terminally ill AIDS patients:

1. Direct lysis of infected cells can be caused by overbearing HIV-1 replication, which can take place upon antigen-specific T-cell activation, hence the term "activation-induced cell death" (Zagury et al. 1986; Cameron et al. 1992).
2. T-cell dysfunction can be brought about by accumulation of multiple copies of unintegrated viral DNA or by toxicity of HIV-encoded proteins (Zack et al. 1990).
3. Syncytium formation is a process by which single infected cells fuse to uninfected cells to form large nonfunctional multinucleated masses (Lifson et al. 1986). These can be readily observed in vitro.
4. Uninfected "bystander" T cells can bind soluble circulating gp120 via their cell-surface CD4 and thus become targeted for killing by gp120-specific cytotoxic T cells (Germain et al. 1988; Siliciano et al. 1988).

5. CD4⁺ T cells from HIV-infected patients undergo spontaneous apoptosis (programed cell death) when treated in vitro with pokeweed mitogen or SEB (Groux et al. 1992). This process is also triggered by cross-linking cell-surface CD4-gp120 complexes with monoclonal antibodies, and by antibodies to TCR components (Banda et al. 1992; Meyaard et al. 1992).

It is clear, however, that none of the above-mentioned mechanisms has yet been proven to act in vivo to such an extent as to be consistent with the massive disappearance of CD4⁺ T cells seen in late phases of HIV disease. Moreover, the frequency of infection of peripheral CD4⁺ T cells in HIV-infected individuals varies between 0.01% and 1%, depending on the detection technique used (Harper et al. 1986; Schnittman et al. 1989). This low frequency is not consistent with lytic destruction of T cells directly resulting from HIV-1 replication. Because HIV-1 is a retrovirus, and since HIV infection, like MMTV *sag*-mediated deletions, implicates CD4⁺ T cells, it was postulated that HIV-1 could encode a gene product with superantigenic properties, which might significantly contribute to the pathogenesis of AIDS (Janeway 1991).

As we have seen, formal demonstration of the presence of a sAg in animal models has relied heavily on revealing specific perturbations in the peripheral TCR Vβ repertoire of affected animals. This repertoire can be typed by a number of methods.

1. Flow cytometric analysis can be performed using panels of monoclonal antibodies directed against each of the 24 Vβ families and numerous subfamilies. Unavailability of complete panels of monoclonal antibodies covering most of the Vβ specificities has so far been the main disadvantage of this procedure.
2. Multiprobe RNase protection assays that employ mixtures of transcripts from cloned TCR Vβ-chain cDNAs have been used in some instances (Baccala et al. 1991). Extensive controls and data correction are required in order to obtain quantitative results.
3. Polymerase chain reaction (PCR) using sets of oligonucleotide primers specific for most of the known Vβ subsets has been used by a number of groups to fingerprint the

expressed Vβ repertoire (Choi et al. 1989; Genevée et al. 1992; Panzara et al. 1992; Soudeyns et al. 1993). The numerous considerations regarding control of amplification specificity, efficacy, and linearity have recently been addressed (Hall and Finn 1992).

Using variations on these methods, Imberti et al. (1991) have shown specific and broad-ranging deletions in the peripheral TCR Vβ repertoire of AIDS patients, but corresponding variations in the TCR Vα repertoire were not seen. Unfortunately, Imberti et al. chose to study patients with advanced HIV disease, who had in some cases experienced multiple opportunistic infections. Thus, they could not adequately control the effects of these opportunistic diseases on the T-cell repertoire. Moreover, whereas v-sAg-mediated T-cell deletions are classically confined to the CD4$^+$ T-cell compartment, these workers performed their typing on total peripheral blood mononuclear cells (PBMC).

Some of these criticisms were addressed by Dalgleish et al. (1992), who typed the Vβ repertoires of asymptomatic HIV-infected individuals, using flow cytometry. Their results suggest that specific expansion of T cells bearing Vβ5.3 determinants is taking place during the course of HIV-1 infection. Unfortunately, the CD4$^+$ T-cell specificity of this putative sAg phenomenon was not addressed. However, the most important objection to these protocols pertains to the fact that study of the human Vβ repertoire must take into account the outbred nature of human populations. Since it has been demonstrated that relative identity between the Vβ repertoires of two given individuals was directly related to the respective likeness of their MHC haplotypes, comparisons between individuals with heterogeneous MHC backgrounds cannot be adequately interpreted, as the great majority of inter-subject variations can be attributed to MHC differences (Gulwani-Akolkar et al. 1991). This problem seriously limits the interpretation of several studies aimed at showing repertoire perturbations in various human illnesses. To take these factors into account, experimental systems developed in our laboratory concentrated on sets of subjects with homologous MHC backgrounds: HIV-1-discordant monozygotic twins; and simulta-

neous typing of various lymphoid compartments within the
same HIV-infected individual.

Vβ REPERTOIRE PERTURBATIONS IN HIV-DISCORDANT MONOZYGOTIC TWINS

It has been demonstrated that the sum of cumulative differences in expression levels of each Vβ chain between two individuals (Δ score) was directly related to the relative difference
in the HLA types of these individuals (Gulwani-Akolkar et al.
1991). Although originally computed starting with flow
cytometric data, this Δ score can also be calculated from
values obtained by quantitative PCR (N. Rebai, unpubl.).
Monozygotic twins display exceedingly similar Vβ repertoires,
perhaps even closer than those of MHC-matched subjects
(D.N. Posnett, pers. comm.; N. Rebai et al., unpubl.). HIV-discordant monozygotic twins therefore represent the ideal system to analyze putative HIV-associated v-sAg effects (Fig. 2).

Using quantitative PCR assay and panels of Vβ-specific
primers, we typed the peripheral Vβ repertoire of 6 pairs of
HIV-discordant monozygotic twins. Subjects ranged in age
from 26 to 40 years old and had CD4 counts ranging from 128
to 1015 cells/mm^3. Furthermore, 4 of 6 subjects had never experienced typical AIDS-associated opportunistic diseases. The
mean Δ score observed in the 6 twin pairs (29.2 ± 11.6; $n = 6$)
was greater than that observed in healthy monozygotic twins
(16.9 ± 3.7; $n = 7$), but lower than that seen in pairs of ran-
domly HLA-mismatched individuals (40.6 ± 7.69; $n = 6$). This
is in agreement with data from Imberti et al. (1991) and Dalgleish et al. (1992), to the extent that it suggests that some
significant perturbation of the TCR Vβ repertoire is ongoing in
HIV-infected patients, whether or not these variations are related to the presence of a v-sAg. Our results further reveal that
significant perturbations in expression of discrete Vβ subsets
(1.5-fold confidence threshold) are restricted to a small, overlapping group of Vβ families: Vβ1 and Vβ21 varied in 3 of 6
cases, Vβ16, -17, and -19 in 2 of 6 cases. Consistent with the
situation seen in murine models, massive deletions of large
fractions of the repertoire were not observed (Fig. 2).

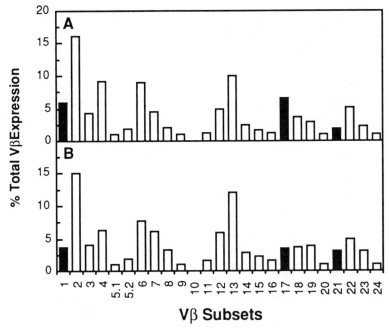

Vβ Subsets

FIGURE 2 This figure represents a comparison between the TCR Vβ repertoire of a representative pair of HIV-discordant monozygotic twins. (A) HIV-negative twin; (B) HIV-positive twin. Expression levels of each Vβ subset were quantitated using PCR and a panel of 24 Vβ-specific oligonucleotides. Briefly, total RNA samples were extracted from PBMC cultures and converted to cDNA using poly(dT)$_{16}$ and AMV reverse transcriptase (Life Sciences, St. Petersburg, Florida). Aliquots of the cDNAs were submitted to 25 cycles of amplification (30 sec/94°, 45 sec/55°, 60 sec/72°) in the GeneAmp PCR system 9600 (Perkin-Elmer Cetus, Emeryville, California), followed by a 7-min/72° extension cycle. Radiolabeled Cβ primer was used as common 3′ primer, and a 200-bp fragment of the Cα gene was also coamplified in each reaction to serve as internal amplification standard. PCR products were separated on 10% polyacrylamide gels (7 M urea), and radioactivity in relevant bands was quantitated using a PhosphorImager (Molecular Dynamics, Sunnyvale, California). Percentage Vβ expression was derived from summation of raw PCR values normalized to the amplification control. By replicate typing, we established that 1.5-fold differences in expression levels represented significant differences (*filled bars*).

Vβ REPERTOIRE PERTURBATIONS BETWEEN LYMPH NODES AND PERIPHERAL BLOOD OF AN HIV-INFECTED SUBJECT

Although most in vivo studies dealing with v-sAgs examine the peripheral Vβ repertoire, only 2% of total body lymphocytes are known to be present in the periphery at any given time. In fact, lymphocyte trafficking is a very dynamic process, as these cells migrate extensively between lymph nodes, spleen, and other lymphoid compartments (for review, see Westermann and Pabst 1990). Moreover, it has been shown that, in HIV-infected patients, the frequency of HIV-infected cells was severalfold greater in lymph nodes than in the periphery, suggesting that these lymphoid compartments bear the bulk of the HIV burden during the course of HIV disease (Pantaleo et al. 1991). We therefore postulated that the most significant Vβ repertoire perturbation would be observed at sites of intense viral replication, namely, within lymph nodes.

We obtained two lymph node biopsies and matching peripheral blood samples from an HIV patient undergoing exploratory surgery for suspected lymphoid malignancies. Results of PCR typing of the Vβ repertoire in respective tissues are shown in Figure 3. Although the patterns of expressed Vβs in both lymph nodes are superimposable, there are twofold and fourfold greater levels of Vβ6- and Vβ21-bearing T cells in the periphery, consistent with deletion of these subsets at sites of intense HIV replication.

IS THERE A v-sAg IN HIV-1 INFECTION?

Other indirect lines of evidence were provided that support the existence of an HIV-associated v-sAg. Laurence et al. (1992) provokingly postulated that if the putative v-sAg played for HIV-1 the same role as the *sag* gene plays for MMTV, namely, to enhance permissiveness for viral replication in specific T-cell subsets, then measurable differences in HIV-1 replication levels should be observed following de novo infection of T-cell clones expressing single TCR Vβ specificities. Indeed, results of such experiments proved that HIV-1 replicated more efficiently in Vβ12-positive than in Vβ6.7a-positive T cells (Laurence et al. 1992). Still, since only Vβ12 and Vβ6.7a were compared, it is unclear whether HIV-1 replication was increased in the former, or decreased in the latter. This could, alternatively, indicate that Vβ6.7a T cells are in fact anergized by the presence of HIV-1, an effect that would be consistent with clinical find-

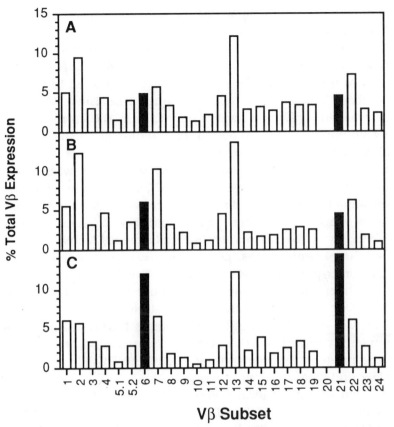

FIGURE 3 Comparison of the Vβ repertoire in peripheral blood and lymph nodes of an HIV-infected individual. This illustrates the percentage expression of each Vβ subset, calculated from quantitative PCR data. (A) Lymph node 1; (B) lymph node 2; (C) peripheral blood. Variations above the 1.5-fold confidence threshold are highlighted (*filled bars*).

ings on activation-induced and programed cell death in lymphocyte cultures from HIV patients (Banda et al. 1992; Meyaard et al. 1992). Unfortunately, typing of HIV-infected individuals failed to demonstrate perturbations in circulating levels of Vβ12- or Vβ6.7a-positive cells (Dalgleish et al. 1992; Laurence et al. 1992). It is therefore of keen interest that our protocols revealed alterations in the levels, and apparent deletion, of Vβ6-expressing T cells in the lymph nodes of an HIV-infected patient (Fig. 3). We are presently investigating this phenomenon by using a Vβ6.7a subfamily-specific probe in PCR typing experiments.

Results from our laboratory have suggested that Vβ repertoire perturbations were taking place during HIV-1 infection, and that these perturbations were restricted to a few Vβ families (Vβ1, -6, -16, -17, -19, and -21). These Vβ chains showed no significant level of homology in the Vβ regions corresponding to those reported to interact with Mls-1a v-sAg (data not shown) (Pullen et al. 1990). Furthermore, deletions were by no means total: This is compatible with murine models of neonatal exogenous MMTV infection, in which only incomplete peripheral disappearance of cognate Vβ subsets takes place (Acha-Orbea and Palmer 1991; Ignatowicz et al. 1992). Even though our typing experiments focused on total peripheral lymphocytes, preliminary results of protocols using cell-sorter-purified CD4$^+$ and CD8$^+$ T cells suggest that the above-mentioned deletions are enhanced in the CD4$^+$ but not the CD8$^+$ compartment (N. Rebai et al., in prep.).

HIV-1 encodes a number of proteins that could potentially possess v-sAg properties. One obvious candidate is the *nef* gene product, a protein whose role in the HIV life cycle is unclear and whose coding sequences, like MMTV *sag*, overlap the 3′ viral LTR (Ahmad and Venkatesan 1988; Kim et al. 1989; Niederman et al. 1992). The viral *env* proteins, gp120 and gp41, are expressed at the cell surface during viral replication; gp120 itself is shed from infected cells into the circulation following CD4 interaction (Hart et al. 1991), a phenomenon thought to be pathogenetically significant (Siliciano et al. 1988). Moreover, *nef*, gp41, and gp120 all display diffuse sequence homology with HLA-DR and -DQ human class II MHC molecules, a finding that potentially reflects distant common ancestry or cryptic functional analogies between these proteins (Golding et al. 1988; Young 1988; Vega et al. 1990). Although no specific interaction between *nef*, *env*, and MHC class II proteins has ever been reported, recent evidence suggests that significant amounts of HLA-DR α and β chains can be found selectively associated with free HIV-1 virions (Arthur et al. 1992). Last, it must be kept in mind that *nef* and *env* proteins are very polymorphic, partly due to the importance of the HIV-1 reverse transcriptase misincorporation rate (Hahn et al.

1986; Preston et al. 1988; Roberts et al. 1988; Meyers et al. 1990; Terwilliger et al. 1991; Shugars et al. 1992). This fact has notable mechanistic implications, since anergy/deletion of a small number of TCR Vβ families by a putative monomorphic HIV-1-encoded v-sAg would be inconsistent with the widespread immune shutdown observed in AIDS patients. Alternatively, polymorphic v-sAg species, whose Vβ specificity varies and evolves during the course of disease progression, could conceivably cause successive obliteration of increasing numbers of CD4$^+$ T-cell subsets.

On the basis of available evidence, which is mostly indirect in nature, we therefore propose the following scheme of v-sAg-induced pathology of HIV-1 infection and AIDS (Fig. 1B): Primary infection of CD4$^+$ cells, be they of lymphocytic, monocytic, or other origin, is followed by release of progeny virions containing HIV-encoded v-sAg of a given initial Vβ specificity. Presentation of this v-sAg to CD4$^+$ T cells, in conjunction with MHC class II, triggers T-cell activation in T-lymphocyte subsets expressing cognate Vβ determinants. As Cameron et al. (1992) demonstrated using cultures of class-II-positive dendritic cells, highly efficient transmission of HIV infection, mediated by cell-to-cell contact, can occur concomitantly with Ag presentation. HIV replication is strongly stimulated by T-cell activation and results in virus-induced cytopathic effects and cell death, as well as in production of new waves of progeny virus. Anergy and deletion then follow in a large proportion of the T-cell subsets reacting with the Vβ-deleting element. New rounds of viral infection and replication give rise to genetic drift of v-sAg Vβ specificity, which can be selectively driven by progressive disappearance of some cellular targets reactive to former v-sAg species. CD4$^+$ T-cell subsets are thus successively anergized and deleted, contributing efficiently to the unrelenting immune failure that heralds terminal HIV disease.

This model of v-sAg function is in large part consistent with that presented for MMTV by Golovkina et al. (1992). A putative HIV-1-associated v-sAg is assimilated to a TCR V-region-specific mitogen that allows high-efficiency viral replication into discrete, activated T-cell subsets. In contrast with MMTV, slow genotypic variations in the HIV-encoded v-sAg could explain sequential activation and deletion of various CD4[+] T-cell subsets, leading to lethal immunosuppression. Furthermore, this model of sAg-mediated HIV pathogenesis does not in any way exclude participation of other established cytopathogenetic mechanisms to the global clinical picture of AIDS.

CONCLUSION

Although superantigens of bacterial and viral origins do not exhibit significant sequence homology, they do share a large spectrum of functional properties. Not only is it clear that both classes of sAg strongly influence immune function, but their relative commonness in the microbial world suggests that there is more to these massive activation phenomena than coincidental interference with normal immune system operations. Indeed, as we have seen exemplified in the study of various viral models, v-sAgs appear in each case to play a role in the life cycles and associated pathogenic processes of their respective viruses, a role significant and dynamic enough to warrant their genetic conservation throughout evolution. Attempts at identifying the specific genes and gene products responsible for these effects are continuing, using in vitro systems and transgenic animals. Therapeutic and immunoprophylactic strategies can potentially be developed to counteract these mechanisms of viral pathogenesis.

ACKNOWLEDGMENTS

The authors thank Dr. H.C. Lane of NIAID, National Institutes of Health, and Dr. J.-P. Routy, Hotel-Dieu de Montréal, for their valuable collaboration on this ongoing project.

REFERENCES

Abe, R. and R.J. Hodes. 1989. T-cell recognition of minor lymphocyte stimulating (Mls) gene products. *Annu. Rev. Immunol.* **7:** 683.

Acha-Orbea, H. and E. Palmer. 1991. Mls-a retrovirus exploits the immune system. *Immunol. Today* **12:** 356.

Ahmad, N. and S. Venkatesan. 1988. Nef protein of HIV-1 is a transcriptional repressor of HIV-1 LTR. *Science* **241:** 1481.

Arthur, L.O., J.W. Bess, Jr., R.C. Sowder II, R.E. Benveniste, D.L. Mann, J.-C. Chermann, and L.E. Henderson. 1992. Cellular proteins bound to immunodeficiency viruses: Implications for pathogenesis and vaccines. *Science* **258:** 1935.

Aziz, D.C., Z. Hanna, and P. Jolicoeur. 1989. Severe immunodeficiency disease induced by a defective murine leukaemia virus. *Nature* **338:** 505.

Baccala, R., D.H. Kono, S. Walker, R.S. Balderas, and A.N. Theofilopoulos. 1991. Genomically imposed and somatically modified human thymocyte Vβ gene repertoires. *Proc. Natl. Acad. Sci.* **88:** 2908.

Baer, G.M. 1988. Animal models in the pathogenesis and treatment of rabies. *Rev. Infect Dis.* **4(S):** 739.

Banda, N.K., J. Bernier, D.K. Kurahara, R. Kurrle, N. Haigwood, R.-P. Sékaly, and T. Helamn Finkel. 1992. Crosslinking CD4 by human immunodeficiency virus gp120 primes T cells for activation-induced apoptosis. *J. Exp. Med.* **176:** 1099.

Behlke, M.A., H.S. Chou, K. Huppi, and D.Y. Loh. 1986. Murine T-cell receptor mutants with deletions of β-chain variable region genes. *Proc. Natl. Acad. Sci.* **83:** 767.

Cameron, P.U., P.S. Freudenthal, J.M. Barker, S. Gezelter, K. Inaba, and R.M. Steinman. 1992. Dendritic cells exposed to human immunodeficiency virus type-1 transmit a vigorous cytopathic infection to CD4+ T cells. *Science* **257:** 383.

Choi, Y., J.W. Kappler, and P. Marrack. 1991. A superantigen encoded in the open reading frame of the 3' long terminal repeat of mouse mammary tumor virus. *Nature* **350:** 203.

Choi, Y., B. Kotzin, L. Herron, J. Callahan, P. Marrack, and J. Kappler. 1989. Interaction of staphylococcus aureus toxin "superantigens" with human T cells. *Proc. Natl. Acad. Sci.* **86:** 8941.

Cole, B.C., and C.L. Atkin. 1991. The mycoplasma arthritidis T-cell mitogen, MAM: A model superantigen. *Immunol. Today* **12:** 271.

Dalgleish, A.G., S. Wilson, M. Gompels, C. Ludlam, B. Gazzard, A.M. Coates, and J. Habeshaw. 1992. T-cell receptor variable gene products and early HIV-1 infection. *Lancet* **339:** 824.

Dewhurst, S., J.E. Embretson, D.C. Anderson, J.I. Mullins, and P.N. Fultz. 1990. Sequence analysis and acute pathogenicity of molecularly cloned $SIV_{SMM-PBj14}$. *Nature* **345:** 636.

Dyson, P.J., A.M. Knight, S. Fairchild, E. Simpson, and K. Tomonari. 1991. Genes encoding ligands for deletion of β11 T cells cosegregate with mammary tumour virus genomes. *Nature* **349:** 531.

Fauci, A.S. 1988. The human immunodeficiency virus: Infectivity and mechanisms of pathogenesis. *Science* **239:** 617.

Fauci, A.S., A.M. Macher, D.L. Longo, H.C. Lane, A.H. Rook, H. Masur, and E.P. Gelmann. 1984. Acquired immunodeficiency syndrome: Epidemiologic, clinical, immunologic and therapeutic considerations. *Ann. Intern Med.* **100:** 92.

Festenstein, H. 1973. Immunogenetics and biological aspects of *in vitro* lymphocyte allotransformation (MLR) in the mouse. *Transplant. Rev.* **15:** 62.

Frankel, W.N., C. Rudy, J.M. Coffin, and B.T. Huber. 1991. Linkage of Mls genes to endogenous mammary tumour viruses of inbred mice. *Nature* **349:** 526.

Fultz, P.N. 1991. Replication of an acutely lethal simian immunodeficiency virus activates and induces proliferation of lymphocytes. *J. Virol.* **65:** 4902.

Gartner, S., P. Markovits, D.M. Markovitz, M.H. Kaplan, R.C. Gallo, and M. Popovic. 1986. The role of mononuclear phagocytes in HTLV-III/LAV infection. *Science* **233:** 215.

Genevée, C., A. Diu, J. Nierat, A. Caignard, P.-Y. Dietrich, L. Ferradini, S. Roman-Roman, F. Triebel, and T. Hercend. 1992. An experimentally validated panel of subfamily-specific oligonucleotide primers (Vα1-w29/Vβ1-w24) for the study of human T cell receptor variable V gene segment usage by polymerase chain reaction. *Eur. J. Immunol.* **22:** 1261.

Germain, R.N. 1988. Antigen processing and CD4$^+$ T cell depletion in AIDS. *Cell* **54:** 441.

Golding, H., F.A. Robey, F.T. Gates III, W. Linder, P.R. Beining, T. Hoffmann, and B. Golding. 1988. Identification of homologous regions in human immunodeficiency virus I gp41 and human MHC class II βI domain. *J. Exp. Med.* **167:** 914.

Golovkina, T.V., A. Chervonsky, J.P. Dudley, and S.R. Ross. 1992. Transgenic mouse mammary tumor virus superantigen expression prevents viral infection. *Cell* **69:** 637.

Groux, H., G. Torpier, D. Monté, Y. Mouton, A. Capron, and J.C. Ameisen. 1992. Activation-induced cell death by apoptosis in CD4$^+$ T cells from human immunodeficiency virus-infected asymptomatic individuals. *J. Exp. Med.* **175:** 331.

Gulwani-Akolkar, B., D.N. Posnett, C.H. Janson, J. Grunewald, H. Wigzell, P. Akolkar, P.K. Gregersen, and J. Silver. 1991. T cell receptor V-segment frequencies in peripheral blood T cells correlate with human leukocyte antigen type. *J. Exp. Med.* **174:** 1139.

Hahn, B.H., G.M. Shaw, M.E. Taylor, R.R. Redfield, P.D. Markham, S. Z. Salahuddin, F. Wong-Staal, R.C. Gallo, E.S. Parks, and W.P. Parks. 1986. Genetic variation in HTLV-III/LAV over time in patients with AIDS or at risk for AIDS. *Science* **232:** 1548.

Hall, B.L. and O.J. Finn. 1992. PCR-based analysis of the T-cell receptor β multigene family: Experimental parameters affecting its validity. *BioTechniques* **13:** 248.

Hanto, D.W., G. Frizzera, K.J. Gajl-Peczalska, and R.L. Simmons. 1985. Epstein-Barr virus, immunodeficiency, and B cell lymphoproliferation. *Transplantation* **39:** 461.

Harper, M.E., L.M. Marselle, R.C. Gallo, and F. Wong-Staal. 1986. Detection of lymphocytes expressing human T-lymphotropic virus type III in lymph nodes and peripheral blood from infected individuals by *in situ* hybridization. *Proc. Natl. Acad. Sci.* **83:** 772.

Hart, T., R. Kirsch, H. Ellens, R. Sweet, D. Lambert, S. Petteway, J. Leary, and P. Bugelski. 1991. Binding of soluble CD4 proteins to HIV-1 and infected cells induces release of envelope glycoprotein gp120. *Proc. Natl. Acad. Sci.* **88:** 2189.

Huang, M. and P. Jolicoeur. 1990. Characterization of the gag fusion protein encoded by the defective Duplan retrovirus inducing murine acquired immunodeficiency syndrome. *J. Virol.* **64:** 5764.

Huang, M., C. Simard, D.G. Kay, and P. Jolicoeur. 1991. The majority of cells infected with the defective murine AIDS virus belong to the B cell lineage. *J. Virol.* **65:** 6562.

Hügin, A.W., M.S. Vacchio, and H.C. Morse III. 1991. A virus-encoded "superantigen" in a retrovirus-induced immunodeficiency syndrome of mice. *Science* **252:** 424.

Ignatowicz, L., J. Kappler, and P. Marrack. 1992. The effects of chronic infection with a superantigen-producing virus. *J. Exp. Med.* **175:** 917.

Imberti, L., A. Sottini, A. Bettinardi, M. Puoti, and D. Primi. 1991. Selective depletion in HIV infection of T cells that bear specific T cell receptor Vβ sequences. *Science* **254:** 860.

Janeway, C.A., J. Yagi, P.J. Conrad, M.E. Katz, B. Jones, S. Vroegop, and S. Buxser. 1989. T-cell responses to Mls and to bacterial proteins that mimic its behavior. *Immunol. Rev.* **107:** 61.

Janeway, C. 1991. Mls: Makes a little sense. *Nature* **349:** 459.

Kanagawa, O., B.A. Nussrallah, M.E. Wiebenga, K.M. Murphy, H.C. Morse III, and F.R. Carbone. 1992. Murine AIDS superantigen reactivity of the T cells bearing Vβ5 T cell antigen receptor. *J. Immunol.* **149:** 9.

Kim, S., K. Ikeuchi, R. Byrn, J. Groopman, and D. Baltimore. 1989. Lack of a negative influence on viral growth by the *nef* gene of human immunodeficiency virus type 1. *Proc. Natl. Acad. Sci.* **86:** 9544.

Klatzmann, D., F. Barre-Sinoussi, M.T. Nugeyre, C. Dauguet, E. Vilmer, C. Griscelli, F. Brun-Vezinet, C. Rouzioux, J.C. Gluckman, J.-C. Chermann, and L. Montagnier. 1984. Selective tropism of lymphadenopathy associated virus (LAV) for helper-inducer T lymphocytes. *Science* **225:** 59.

Kubo, Y., Y. Nakagawa, K. Kakimi, H. Matsui, M. Iwashiro, K. Kuribayashi, T. Masuda, H. Hiai, T. Hirama, S.-I. Yanagawa, and A. Ishimoto. 1992. Presence of transplantable T-lymphoid cells in C57BL/6 mice infected with murine AIDS virus. *J. Virol.* **66:** 5691.

Lafon, M., M. Lafage, A. Martinez-Arends, R. Ramirez, F. Vuillier, D. Charron, V. Lotteau, and D. Scott-Algara. 1992. Evidence for a viral superantigen in humans. *Nature* **358:** 507.

Laurence, J., A.S. Hodtsev, and D.N. Posnett. 1992. Superantigen implicated in dependence of HIV-1 replication in T cells on TCR Vβ expression. *Nature* **358:** 255.

Legrand, E., R. Daluculsi, and J.F. Duplan. 1981. Characteristics of the cell populations involved in extra-thymic lymphosarcoma induced in C57BL/6 mice by RadLV-Rs. *Leuk. Res.* **5:** 223.

Lifson, J.D., M.B. Feinberg, G.R. Reyes, L. Rabin, B. Banapour, S. Chakrabarti, B. Moss, F. Wong-Staal, K.S. Steimer, and E.G. Engleman. 1986. Induction of CD4-dependent cell fusion by the HTLV-III/LAV envelope glycoprotein. *Nature* **323:** 725.

Maddon, P.J., A.G. Dalgleish, J.S. McDougal, P.R. Clapham, R.A. Weiss, and R. Axel. 1986. The T4 gene encodes the AIDS virus receptor and is expressed in the immune system and the brain. *Cell* **47:** 333.

Marrack, P. and J. Kappler. 1990. The staphylococcal enterotoxins and their relatives. *Science* **248:** 705.

Marrack, P., E. Kushnir, and J. Kappler. 1991. A maternally inherited superantigen encoded by a mammary tumour virus. *Nature* **349:** 524.

Meyaard, L., S.A. Otto, R.R. Jonker, M.J. Mijnster, R.P.M. Keet, and F. Miedema. 1992. Programmed death of T cells in HIV-1 infection. *Science* **257:** 217.

Meyers, G., A.B. Rabson, J.A. Berzofsky, F.T. Smith, and F. Wong-Staal, eds. 1990. *Human retroviruses and AIDS: A compilation and analysis of nucleic acid and amino acid sequences.* Los Alamos National Laboratory, New Mexico.

Monroe, J.E., A. Calender, and C. Mulder. 1988. Epstein-Barr virus-positive and -negative B-cell lines can be infected with human immunodeficiency virus types 1 and 2. *J. Virol.* **62:** 3497.

Moore, R., M. Dixon, R. Smith, G. Peters, and C. Dickson. 1987. Complete nucleotide sequence of a milk-transmitted mouse mammary tumor virus: Two frameshift suppression events are required for translation of *gag* and *pol. J. Virol.* **61:** 480.

Mosier, D.E., R.A. Yetter, and H.C. Morse III. 1985. Retroviral induction of acute lymphoproliferative disease and profound immunosuppression in C57BL/10 mice. *J. Exp. Med.* **161:** 766.

Niederman, T.M. J., J.V. Garcia, W.R. Hastings, S. Luria, and L. Ratner. 1992. Human immunodeficiency virus type 1 nef protein inhibits NF-κB induction in human T cells. *J. Virol.* **66:** 6213.

Okada, Y., K. Suzuki, K. Komuro, and T. Mizuochi. 1992. High frequency of transmission of murine AIDS virus in C57BL/10 mice *via* mother's milk. *J. Virol.* **66:** 5177.

Pantaleo, G., C. Graziosi, L. Butini, P.A. Pizzo, S.M. Schnittman, D.P. Kotler, and A.S. Fauci. 1991. Lymphoid organs function as major reservoirs for human immunodeficiency virus. *Proc. Natl. Acad. Sci.* **88:** 9838.

Panzara, M.A., E. Gussoni, L. Steinman, and J.R. Oksenberg. 1992. Analysis of the T cell repertoire using PCR and specific oligonucleotide primers. *BioTechniques* **12:** 728.

Perry, L.L., and D.L. Lodmell. 1991. Role of CD4$^+$ and CD8$^+$ T cells in murine resistance to street rabies virus. *J. Virol.* **65:** 3429.

Perry, L.L., J.D. Hotchkiss, and D.L. Lodmell. 1990. Murine susceptibility to street rabies virus is unrelated to induction of host lymphoid depletion. *J. Immunol.* **144:** 3552.

Preston, B.D., B.J. Poiesz, and L.A. Loeb. 1988. Fidelity of HIV-1 reverse transcriptase. *Science* **242:** 1168.

Pullen, A.M., T. Wade, P. Marrack, and J. Kappler. 1990. Identification of the region of T cell receptor β chain that interacts with the self-superantigen Mls-1a. *Cell* **61:** 1365.

Pullen, A.M., J. Bill, R.T. Kubo, P. Marrack, and J.W. Kappler. 1991. Analysis of the interaction site for the self superantigen Mls-1a on T cell receptor Vβ. *J. Exp. Med.* **173:** 1183.

Roberts, J.D., K. Bebenek, and T.A. Kunkel. 1988. The accuracy of reverse transcriptase from HIV-1. *Science* **242:** 1171.

Salmons, B. and W.H. Gunzburg. 1987. Current perspectives in the biology of mouse mammary tumour virus. *Virus Res.* **8:** 81.

Schnittman, S.M., M.C. Psallidopoulos, H.C. Lane, L. Thompson, M. Baseler, F. Massari, C.H. Fox, N.P. Salzman, and A.S. Fauci. 1989. The reservoir for HIV-1 in human peripheral blood is a T cell that maintains expression of CD4. *Science* **245:** 305.

Shugars, D.C., D. Glueck, and R. Swanstrom. 1992. Sequence heterogeneity of the HIV-1 *nef* gene. *J. Cell. Biochem.* **S16E:** 41.

Siliciano, R.F., T. Lawton, C. Knall, R.W. Karr, P. Berman, T. Gregory, and E.L. Reinherz. 1988. Analysis of host-virus interactions in AIDS with anti-gp120 T cell clones: Effect of HIV sequence variation and a mechanism for CD4$^+$ cell depletion. *Cell* **54:** 561.

Simard, C. and P. Jolicoeur. 1991. The effect of anti-neoplastic drugs on murine acquired immunodeficiency syndrome. *Science* **251:** 305.

Soudeyns, H., N. Rebai, G.P. Pantaleo, C. Ciurli, T. Boghossian, R.-P. Sékaly, and A.S. Fauci. 1993. The T cell receptor Vβ repertoire in HIV-1 infection and disease. *Semin. Immunol.* **5:** 175.

Sugamata, M., M. Myazawa, S. Mori, G.J. Spangrude, L.C. Ewalt, and D.L. Lodmell. 1992. Paralysis of street rabies virus-infected mice is dependent on T lymphocytes. *J. Virol.* **66:** 1252.

Terwilliger, E.F., E. Langhoff, D. Gabuzda, E. Zazopoulos, and W.A. Haseltine. 1991. Allelic variation in the effects of the *nef* gene on replication of human immunodeficiency virus type 1. *Proc. Natl. Acad. Sci.* **88:** 10971.

Thomson, B.J. and J. Nicholas. 1991. Superantigen function. *Nature* **351:** 530.

Torres-Anjel, M.J., D. Volz, M.J. Torres, M. Turk, and J.G. Tshikuka. 1988. Failure to thrive, wasting syndrome, and immunodeficiency in rabies: A hypophyseal/hypothalamic/thymic axis effect of rabies virus. *Rev. Infect Dis.* (suppl.)**10:** S710.

Vega, M.A., R. Guigó, and T.F. Smith. 1990. Autoimmune response in AIDS. *Nature* **345:** 26.

Westermann, J. and R. Pabst. 1990. Lymphocyte subsets in the blood: A diagnostic window on the lymphoid system? *Immunol. Today* **11:** 406.

Woodland, D.L., M.P. Happ, K.J. Gollob, and E. Palmer. 1991. An endogenous retrovirus mediating deletion of αβ T cells? *Nature* **349:** 529.

Young, J.A.T. 1988. HIV and HLA similarity. *Nature* **333:** 215.

Zack, J.A., S.J. Arrigo, S.R. Weitsman, A.S. Go, A. Haislip, and I.Y. Chen. 1990. HIV-1 entry into quiescent primary lymphocytes: Molecular analysis reveals a labile, latent viral structure. *Cell* **61:** 213.

Zagury, D., J. Bernard, R. Leonard, R. Cheynier, M. Feldman, P.S. Sarin, and R.C. Gallo. 1986. Long-term cultures of HTLV-III-infected T cells: A model of cytopathology of T-cell depletion in AIDS. *Science* **231:** 850.

HIV-1 Replication in T Cells Dependent on TCR Vβ Expression

D.N. Posnett, S. Kabak, A. Asch, and A.S. Hodtsev

Divisions of Allergy/Immunology and Hematology/Oncology, Department of Medicine, Cornell University Medical College, New York, New York 10021

A superantigen (sAg) appears to play an important role in establishing infection by the exogenous mouse mammary tumor viruses (MMTV) (Acha-Orbea and Palmer 1991; Coffin 1992; Golovkina et al. 1992). The sAg is encoded by the 3′ LTR ORF gene (Acha-Orbea et al. 1991; Choi et al. 1991). If the sAg-reactive T cells are functionally deleted as in sAg transgenic mice (Golovkina et al. 1992), viral infection is highly inefficient. Presumably, this is because the virus now lacks a mechanism to activate host lymphoid cells, in which it may replicate and establish a latent reservoir.

The findings with MMTV could serve as a model for HIV-1 infection. As a test of this hypothesis, we obtained evidence for Vβ-selective HIV-1 replication both in vitro and in vivo, which is summarized herein. Possible sources of an HIV-1-associated sAg and the potential significance of a sAg in HIV-1 infection are discussed. Since the HIV-1-associated sAg has not yet been identified at the molecular level, we prefer to make no assumptions about the molecular size and nature of the putative "superantigen" and use this term only in the sense of "Vβ-selective element" (Janeway 1991).

HIV-1 REPLICATION IN Vβ-SELECTED CELL LINES

T-cell lines expressing selected Vβ T-cell receptor (TCR) gene products were produced from normal donors. Fresh peripheral blood lymphocytes (PBL) were used for positive selection with Vβ-specific monoclonal antibodies and goat anti-mouse

Superantigens: A Pathogen's View of the Immune System

Ig-coated magnetic beads. Selected T cells were then expanded with 5% IL-2 containing medium and Na-periodate-treated allogeneic feeder cells added to the cultures about every 10 days. Such cell lines become more than 95% enriched for T cells expressing the selected Vβ over 2–3 weeks (Posnett et al. 1988; Laurence et al. 1992). Cell lines derived in parallel from the same blood sample were used in all experiments. These cell lines were always treated in exactly the same way and had very similar baseline proliferative characteristics (Fig. 1), as well as similar expression of surface activation antigens and adhesion molecules, including CD4 and CD8 (Fig. 2) (Laurence et al. 1992). They were therefore felt to be comparable in terms of their ability to act as host cells for HIV-1 replication. They

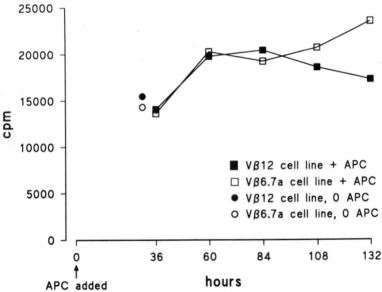

FIGURE 1 Baseline ^{3}H-thymidine incorporation for a set of Vβ-selected cell lines. A Vβ6.7a cell line and a Vβ12 cell line (>95% cells express the selected Vβ) were derived in parallel from the same blood sample. After two cycles (14 days) of weekly feeding with periodate-treated non-T-cells (denoted APC) and maintenance in 5% IL-2-containing medium, the cells were split and either cultured without further additives for 36 hr (circles) or admixed with 20% irradiated APCs and cultured for various time periods. A 12-hr ^{3}H-thymidine pulse was used to determine DNA synthesis at the indicated time points.

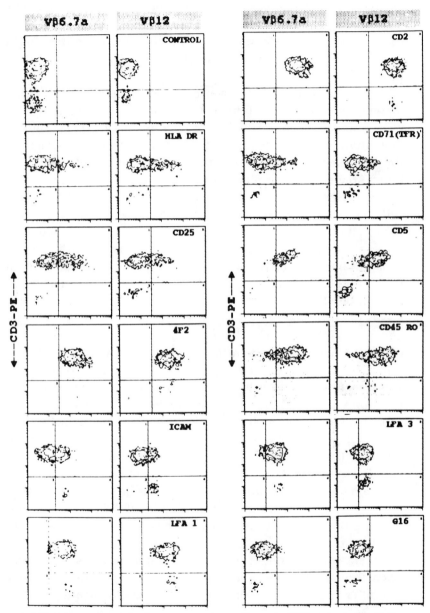

FIGURE 2 Phenotypic characterization of a set of Vβ-selected cell lines. The two cell lines described in Fig. 1 were stained by two-color immunofluorescence with anti-CD3-PE (*ordinate*) and various indicated activation antigens indirectly labeled with GAM-FITC (*abscissa*). G16 is an unpublished activation antigen of lymphocytes.

clearly represented partially activated (IL-2R⁺, HLA-DR⁺) T cells and not resting T cells. These sets of cell lines were used to measure and compare HIV-1 replication (p24 capture ELISA assay, or reverse transcriptase [RT] assay) at multiple time points.

Using the isolate TIIIB, we found HIV-1 replication varied among different Vβ cell lines (Laurence et al. 1992). HIV-1 replication was often 100-fold greater in Vβ12-expressing cell lines than in Vβ6.7a cell lines, regardless of the donor-origin of the cell lines. Because replication differed most between Vβ12 and Vβ6.7a cells, we focused on comparisons between these two Vβ subsets. HIV-1 replication was restricted to the CD4 cells in these cultures. No viral replication was observed when CD4 cells were removed, but replication was not affected by removal of CD8 cells. Addition of MHC class-II-positive feeder cells (prepared as mentioned above) was necessary for optimal HIV-1 replication in CD4⁺ Vβ12⁺ T cells, and replication could be inhibited by 80% using a cocktail of five anti-class-II monoclonal antibodies added to the cultures. These features, as well as the lack of differences observed between cell lines derived from HLA disparate donors, suggested that HIV-1 might be associated with expression of a non-HLA-restricted sAg targeting Vβ12 T cells. Consistent with this interpretation, we found that Vβ6.7a T cells could be activated to serve as good host cells for high-level HIV-1 replication, as seen with the Vβ12 cells. This was achieved by adding PHA + PMA to the cultures (Laurence et al. 1992) or by addition of exogenous sAg, such as TSST-1 or SEE, which can activate Vβ6.7a T cells (D.N. Posnett, unpubl.). Moreover, a small level of HIV-1 replication can always be appreciated in Vβ6.7a cells (without the addition of mitogens or exogenous sAg) (Laurence et al. 1992), and viral cDNA can be found in these cells by polymerase chain reaction (PCR) with *gag* primers. This suggests that the host cells are equivalent in terms of viral entry but differ in the support of intracellular viral replication.

Vβ TROPISM OF DIFFERENT HIV-1 ISOLATES

Of interest was the degree of replication observed in these cell lines with HIV-1 isolates other than TIIIB. To date, we have

reproducible data with BAL (Laurence et al. 1992) and the
street isolate MART (D.N. Posnett and J. Laurence, unpubl.),
both of which replicate better in Vβ12 than in Vβ6.7a cell
lines. However, the RF isolate gives different results. Here viral
replication is usually higher and occurs earlier in Vβ6.7a cells
than in Vβ12 cells (Fig. 3). These data suggest that different
HIV-1 isolates may be associated with sAg of varying Vβ target
specificity. Such a system would closely resemble the large
number of different specificities encoded by the sAg of the
MMTVs (Acha-Orbea and Palmer 1991), which are thought to
have evolved in order for MMTV to assure its survival in
murine hosts that have deleted targeted Vβ subsets (Coffin
1992). The findings with the RF isolate also provide an experimental approach to identifying the HIV-1 gene product which

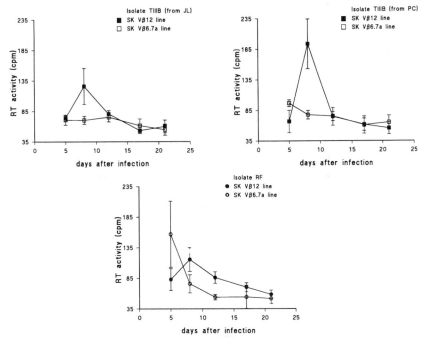

FIGURE 3 TIIIB and RT HIV-1 isolates have different Vβ-selective
replication patterns. A set of Vβ-selected cell lines was used for in
vitro infection with 1000 TCID of two preparations of TIIIB (prepared
in two different laboratories) or 1000 TCID of the RT isolate. HIV-1
replication was determined using an RT assay (Cameron et al. 1992).
Culture conditions were otherwise as stated by Laurence et al. (1992).

may act as a sAg. This can be done by constructing hybrid viral strains, part TIIIB and part RF, and measuring replication in Vβ12 and Vβ6.7a cell lines.

Vβ-SELECTIVE PROLIFERATION INDUCED BY PATIENT-DERIVED NON-T-CELLS

Known sAg invariably cause T-cell proliferation when the purified sAg are added to in vitro cultures. This is less readily apparent when unpurified bacterial or mycoplasma culture supernatants are used as a source of sAg (Atkin et al. 1986). In the case of the HIV-1-associated sAg, purified material is not available, and culture supernatants of HIV-1-infected cells are known to contain inhibitory factors for T-cell proliferation (Levy 1993). Moreover, soluble and cell-bound env gene products may bind to CD4 and elicit a negative signal (Biddison et al. 1982; Bank and Chess 1985), result in syncitium formation, or result in apoptotic CD4 T-cell death (Banda et al. 1992). This may explain why HIV-1-containing supernatants and recombinant gp120/gp160 preparations are not mitogenic for fresh human T cells in our hands (D.N. Posnett, unpubl.).

We therefore chose to analyze antigen-presenting non-T-cells from HIV-1-seropositive hemophiliac patients as a source of the putative HIV-1-associated sAg (Laurence et al. 1992). By analogy with MMTV sAg, which are expressed in the mouse by activated B cells, we used the non-T-cell fraction of peripheral blood mononuclear cells, which would include B cells, monocytes, and dendritic cells, all capable of presenting exogenous sAg, like the staphylococcal enterotoxins, to T cells (Bhardwaj et al. 1992). These cells were irradiated and cocultured with allogeneic T cells. However, large numbers of stimulator cells were necessary to observe T-cell proliferation of fresh resting T cells, making it difficult to discern between alloreactivity and the putative sAg reactivity. When Vβ-selected cell lines were utilized (prepared as described above), proliferation of T cells was readily observed using smaller numbers of stimulator cells (1:1 or 1:3 ratio of stimulators to T cells) after 3 days of culture (Laurence et al. 1992). Under these conditions, no allo-responses were observed, since control allogeneic stimulator cells from HIV-1-negative donors failed to induce proliferation of either Vβ12⁺ or Vβ6.7a⁺ cell lines. In contrast, anti-CD3 monoclonal antibody induced proliferation of both cell lines. Stimulator non-T-cells from 5 of 8 HIV-1-seropositive hemophiliac patients selectively induced proliferation of the Vβ12 cells and not the Vβ6.7a cells (Laurence et al. 1992). Therefore, these data are consistent with expression of a sAg-like molecule on a subset of non-T-cells from HIV-1-infected patients.

LACK OF PREFERENTIAL DELETION OF Vβ SUBSETS IN AIDS

It has been suggested that an HIV-1-associated sAg may in part cause the progressive depletion of CD4⁺ cells in AIDS by inducing apoptosis of targeted Vβ subsets (Groux et al. 1991). However, it makes little teleological sense that a virus would induce the depletion of the very cells it prefers to replicate in. The model of exogenous milk-borne MMTV in C3H mice indicates that the primary purpose of this virally encoded sAg is to assure an early peak of viral replication by activating CD4⁺ host cells (Acha-Orbea and Palmer 1991; Held et al. 1993; Waanders et al. 1993). Thus, HIV-1 may activate selected Vβ subsets to promote initial viral replication and establish a viral reservoir in these subsets. To examine the issue of Vβ-selective CD4 T-cell depletion, we used two-color fluorescence with CD4 and CD8 monoclonal antibody conjugated to phycoerythrin and 11 TCR V-gene-specific monoclonal antibodies, marked indirectly with FITC (Posnett et al. 1993a). In samples taken from 44 HIV-1-seropositive hemophiliac patients, percentages of T-cells expressing Vβ12, Vβ6.7a, Vβ8, Vβ17, Vβ5.1, Vβ5.2/3, Vβ13.3, Vβ3, Vα2.3, and Vα12.1 were similar to those in normal controls (Posnett et al. 1993a). These results were also valid in comparisons with patients in different clinical stages of disease. Vβ expression did not correlate with total numbers of CD4 cells in these patients. Thus, in this population of unrelated patients, no Vβ-selective T-cell depletion was observed. These results fail to confirm a previous study in which Vβ subsets were measured by RT-PCR and in which Vβ17 T cells (among others) were reported to be absent in AIDS patients (Imberti et al. 1991). Our negative results may relate to the large polymorphism of HIV-1 isolates found in patients, in particular those who have harbored virus for prolonged periods (Starcich et al. 1986; Fisher et al. 1988; Pang et al. 1992; Wolinsky et al. 1992), like the hemophilia patients, who were all infected prior to 1984. Perhaps the various viral isolates have different Vβ-specific replication patterns, as suggested by the studies on 4 isolates described above. In vivo, a large array of different viral isolates could cancel out any specific Vβ deletion due to a single isolate. This possibility is difficult to rule out at the present time, but the finding that HIV-1 viral DNA is preferentially distributed in Vβ12 cells (see below) and the Vβ-selective stimulation obtained with non-T-cells from seropositive patients (see above) both suggest that a Vβ12-selective element is operative in vivo and that its effects can be detected despite the large number of polymorphic isolates.

BIASED DISTRIBUTION OF HIV-1 DNA AMONG Vβ T-CELL SUBSETS

To measure viral load in different Vβ subsets, a quantitative PCR method was used with dilutions of the ACH2 cell line to construct a standard curve. This cell line carries a single non-productive integrated copy of viral DNA per genome. Therefore, known dilutions of these cells with uninfected cells provide a known number of viral DNA copies per PCR reaction. Typically, the PCR assay detects 1–10 viral DNA copies using a set of *gag* primers corresponding to conserved sequences, one of which is end-labeled with [32]P. As an internal control for the total amount of cellular DNA in the PCR reaction, we include a set of HLA-DQα primers in the same reaction. Dilutions of total numbers of T cells tested with the HLA-DQ primers provide a standard curve for estimating the numbers of cells in the experimental samples.

Using monoclonal antibodies specific for Vβ12, Vβ6.7a, and in some cases Vβ8, Vβ17, and Vβ3, we have isolated these Vβ subsets by positive selection using goat anti-mouse-coated magnetic beads. The cells are immediately lysed while still adherent to the magnetic beads, and DNA is extracted and used as substrate in the PCR reaction. HIV-1 load was quantitated in Vβ12 and Vβ6.7a subsets in 22 seropositive hemophilia patients (Posnett et al. 1993b). In 13 patients (59%), the ratio of HIV-1 load in Vβ12/Vβ6.7a cells was greater than 3 (range 3–34.5). In 7 patients (32%), the ratio was mildly skewed to Vβ12 cells (range 1–3), and in 2 patients (9%) the HIV-1 load was greater in Vβ6.7a cells than in Vβ12 cells (ratio 0.3 and 0.6). Clinical criteria of disease such as the presence of opportunistic infections and "clinical AIDS" or the total CD4 count did not correlate with the ratio of HIV load in the 2 Vβ subsets. A mild correlation of advanced disease (clinical AIDS and CD4 count below 200/μl) with high total HIV load (viral copies/1000 T cells) was observed, consistent with prior observations (Schnittman et al. 1989; Bagasra et al. 1992; Piatak et al. 1993; Patterson et al. 1993). These patient data represent an independent confirmation of the in vitro studies showing high-level HIV-1 replication in Vβ12 cells and suggest that this phenomenon is relevant to in vivo infection in man. The data do not distinguish between different multiplicities of infection. In situ PCR (Bagasra et al. 1992; Patterson et al. 1993) will be required to accurately count the numbers of Vβ12 and Vβ6.7a cells that contain HIV-1 DNA. The data also do not distinguish between cells capable of producing infectious virions and cells harboring defective virus. This is an important point, since a viral "reservoir" (e.g., sAg-targeted Vβ12 cells) should be capable of producing infectious virus; current estimates of the in vivo ratio of infectious virus per total viral load are 1:60,000 (Piatak et al. 1993).

DISCUSSION

Several observations indicate that the HIV-1 virus is not very efficient in establishing infection when transmitted via blood products from a donor to a recipient. First, the incidence of infection after accidental exposure is at least tenfold less than with hepatitis B and C viruses (Gibbons et al. 1990). Second, there are well-described cases of hemophiliac patients who repeatedly received contaminated lots of factor VIII prior to 1986 and yet remained uninfected, as assessed by PCR (Gibbons et al. 1990). Among HIV-1-exposed individuals who fail to seroconvert, approximately 50% exhibit cell-mediated immunity to HIV gp160 peptides in vitro, indicating that these patients were exposed to HIV-1 but did not become infected. These patients include homosexuals with known exposure, health care workers exposed by accidental needle sticks, and newborn infants of seropositive mothers (Clerici et al. 1991, 1992; Salk et al. 1993). Moreover, it is now clear that the majority of babies born to HIV-seropositive mothers do not seroconvert and remain PCR-negative for HIV-1 with follow-up periods of several years (Brandt et al. 1992). The in vitro corollary is the well-established observation that it is difficult to infect resting T cells without the addition of mitogens to activate them in culture (McDougal et al. 1985).

Transmission from one host to another therefore appears to be a critical period during which the virus could benefit from optimal activation of host cells in which to replicate. A high level of initial replication would assure transmission to a large number of host cells, and this probably occurs during the first weeks after exposure, during the clinically acute phase of infection associated with high levels of viremia (Clark et al. 1991; Daar et al. 1991). After this acute phase, some latently infected cells may be difficult to eradicate because integrated viral DNA is minimally expressed. Such cells seem to evade the immune system and ensure low-grade persistent viral infection. This would provide the virus with sufficient time to infect new human hosts.

In vivo, efficient activation of targeted T cells could occur when HIV-1 (or HIV-1-derived antigen) is "presented" to T cells via dendritic cells (Cameron et al. 1992). Alternatively, HIV-1 might encode a potent sAg that would be able to activate targeted T cells for maximal viral replication (Laurence et al. 1992). A possible scenario is that a component of gp160 represents the Vβ-selective element, as depicted in Figure 4. A deviation on this theme is that HIV-1 activates human host cells to express an endogenous superantigen (Table 1). The latter has not yet been described, but one might speculate that any of numerous retroviral sequences contained in the human genome could encode a superantigen, in a manner analogous to endogenous MMTVs in mice, or that ubiquitous viruses that infect most humans, like Epstein-Barr virus, could encode a usually nonexpressed superantigen.

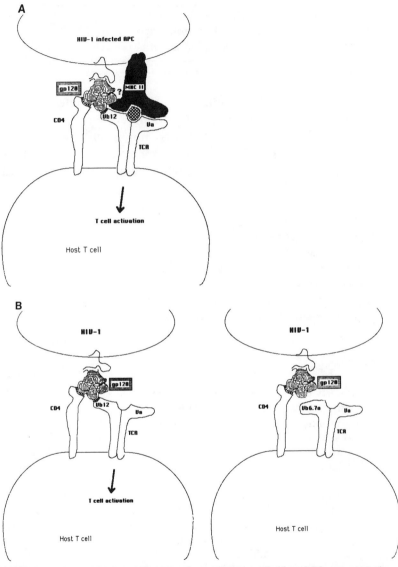

FIGURE 4 (*A*) Possible scenario if a component of gp160 represents a Vβ-selective element or sAg. A crucial question is whether binding to class II MHC can be demonstrated or not. (*B*) HIV-1 virions themselves may activate targeted host T cells (such as Vβ12 cells), since they may express surface class II molecules derived from host cell membranes at the time of viral budding (Arthur et al. 1992). The latter are not depicted in *B* for the sake of clarity.

TABLE 1 *POSSIBLE SOURCES OF HIV-ASSOCIATED SAG*

1. Encoded by HIV-1 gene (gp160, nef, etc.)
2. Encoded by alternative ubiquitous virus (EBV, CMV)
3. Encoded by host cell gene (endogenous retroviral sequences)

It is important to understand the sAg-like effects described herein, because prevention of acute HIV infection could involve some balance of inhibition of early nonspecific immune activation (e.g., via sAg) and enhancement of a specific immune response involving both cytotoxic T lymphocytes and antibody responses.

ACKNOWLEDGMENTS

This work was funded in part by RO-1-AI33322-01 and by a fellowship award from the Aaron Diamond Foundation to A.S.H. The viral isolates were kindly provided by Drs. J. Laurence and P. Cameron.

REFERENCES

Acha-Orbea, H. and E. Palmer. 1991. Mls—A retrovirus exploits the immune system. *Immunol. Today* **12:** 356.

Acha-Orbea, H., A.N. Shakov, L. Scarpellino, E. Kolb, V. Müller, A. Vessaz-Shaw, R. Fuchs, K. Blöchinger, P. Rollini, J. Billotte, M. Sarafidou, H.R. MacDonald, and H. Diggelmann. 1991. Clonal deletion of Vβ14-bearing T cells in mice transgenic for mammary tumour virus. *Nature* **350:** 207.

Arthur, L.O., Jr. J.W. Bess, R.C. Sowder II, R.E. Benveniste, D.L. Mann, J.-C. Chermann, and L.E. Henderson. 1992. Cellular proteins bound to immunodeficiency viruses: Implications for pathogenesis and vaccines. *Science* **258:** 1935.

Atkin, C.L., B.C. Cole, G.J. Sullivan, L.R. Washburn, and B.B. Wiley. 1986. Stimulation of mouse lymphocytes by a mitogen derived from *Mycoplasma arthritidis*. V. A small basic protein from culture supernatants is a potent T cell mitogen. *J. Immunol.* **137:** 1581.

Bagasra, O., S.P. Hauptman, H.W. Lischner, M. Sachs, and R.J. Pomerantz. 1992. Detection of human immunodeficiency virus type 1 provirus in mononuclear cells by in situ polymerase chain reaction. *N. Engl. J. Med.* **326:** 1385.

Banda, N.K., J. Bernier, D.K. Kurahara, R. Kurrle, N. Haigwood, R-P.

Sekaly, and T.H. Finkel. 1992. Crosslinking CD4 by HIV gp120 primes T cells for activation-induced apoptosis. *J. Exp. Med.* **176:** 1099.

Bank, I. and L. Chess. 1985. Perturbation of the T4 molecule transmits a negative signal to T cells. *J. Exp. Med.* **162:** 1294.

Bhardwaj, N., S.M. Friedman, B.C. Cole, and A.J. Nisanian. 1992. Dendritic cells are potent antigen-presenting cells for microbial superantigens. *J. Exp. Med.* **175:** 267.

Biddison, W.E., P.E. Rao, M.A. Talle, G. Goldstein, and S. Shaw. 1982. Possible involvement of the OKT4 molecule in T cell recognition of class II HLA antigens. *J. Exp. Med.* **156:** 1065.

Brandt, C.D., T.A. Rakusan, A.V. Sison, S.H. Josephs, E.S Saxena, K.D. Herzog, R.H. Parrott, and J.L. Sever. 1992. Detection of human immunodeficiency virus type 1 infection in young pediatric patients by using polymerase chain reaction and biotinylated probes. *J. Clin. Microbiol.* **30:** 36.

Cameron, P.U., P.S. Freudenthal, J.M. Barker, S. Gezelter, K. Inaba, and R.M. Steinman. 1992. Dendritic cells exposed to human immunodeficiency virus type-1 transmit a vigorous cytopathic infection to CD4+ T cells. *Science* **257:** 383.

Choi, Y., J.W. Kappler, and P. Marrack. 1991. A superantigen encoded in the open reading frame of the 3' long terminal repeat of mouse mammary tumour virus. *Nature* **350:** 203.

Clark, S.J., M.S. Saag, W.D. Decker, S. Campbell-Hill, J.L. Roberson, P.J. Veldkamp, J.C. Kappes, B.H. Hahn, and G.M. Shaw. 1991. High titers of cytopathic virus in plasma of patients with symptomatic primary HIV-1 infection. *N. Engl. J. Med.* **324:** 954.

Clerici, M., J.A. Berzofsky, G.M. Shearer, and C.O. Tacket. 1991. Exposure to human immunodeficiency virus type-1 specific T helper cell responses before detection of infection by polymerase chain reaction and serum antibodies. *J. Infect. Dis.* **164:** 178.

Clerici, M., J.V. Giorgi, C-C. Chou, V.K. Gudeman, J.A. Zack, P. Gupta, H-N. Ho, P.G. Nishanaian, J.A. Berzofsky, and G.M. Shearer. 1992. Cell-mediated immune response to human immunodeficiency virus (HIV) type-1 in seronegative homosexual men with recent sexual exposure to HIV-1. *J. Infect. Dis.* **165:** 1012.

Coffin, J.M. 1992. Superantigens and endogenous retroviruses: A confluence of puzzles. *Science* **255:** 411.

Daar, E.S., T. Moudgil, D. Meyer, and D.D. Ho. 1991. Transient high levels of viremia in patients with primary human immunodeficiency virus type 1 infection. *N. Engl. J. Med.* **324:** 961.

Fisher, A.G., B. Ensoli, D. Looney, A. Rose, R.C. Gallo, M.S. Saag, G.M. Shaw, B.H. Hahn, and F. Wong-Staal. 1988. Biologically diverse molecular variants within a single HIV-1 isolate. *Nature* **334:** 444.

Gibbons, J., J.M. Cory, I.K. Hewlett, J.S. Epstein, and M.E. Eyster.

1990. Silent infections with human immunodeficiency virus type 1 are highly unlikely in multitransfused seronegative hemophiliacs. *Blood* **76:** 1924.

Golovkina, T.V., A. Chervonsky, J.P. Dudley, and S.R. Ross. 1992. Transgenic mouse mammary tumor virus superantigen expression prevents viral infection. *Cell* **69:** 637.

Groux, H., G. Torpier, D. Monte, Y. Mouton, A. Capron, and J.C. Ameisen. 1991. Activation-induced death by apoptosis in CD4⁺ T cells from HIV-infected asymptomatic individuals. *J. Exp. Med.* **175:** 331.

Held, W., A.N. Shakhov, S. Izui, G.A. Waanders, L. Scarpellino, H.R. MacDonald, and H. Acha-Orbea. 1993. Superantigen-reactive CD4⁺ T cells are required to stimulate B cells after infection with mouse mammary tumor virus. *J. Exp. Med.* **177:** 359.

Imberti, L., A. Sottini, A. Bettinardi, M. Puoti, and D. Primi. 1991. Selective depletion in HIV infection of T cells that bear specific T cell receptor Vβ sequences. *Science* **254:** 860.

Janeway, C.A. 1991. Immune recognition: Mls—Makes little sense. *Nature* **349:** 459.

Laurence, J., A.S. Hodtsev, and D.N. Posnett. 1992. Superantigen implicated in dependence of HIV-1 replication in T cells on TCR Vβ expression. *Nature* **358:** 255.

Levy, J. 1993. Pathogenesis of human immunodeficiency virus infection. *Microbiol. Rev.* **57:** 183.

McDougal, J.S., A. Mawle, S.P. Cort, J.K.A. Nicholson, G.D. Cross, J.A. Scheppler-Campbell, D. Hicks, and J. Sligh. 1985. Cellular tropism of the human retrovirus, HTLV-III/LAV. I. Role of T cell activation and expression of the T4 antigen. *J. Immunol.* **135:** 3151.

Pang, S., Y. Shlesinger, E.S. Daar, T. Moudgil, D.D. Ho, and I.S. Chen. 1992. Rapid generation of sequence variation during primary HIV-1 infection. *AIDS* **6:** 453.

Patterson, B.K., M. Till, P. Otto, C. Goolsby, M.R. Furtado, L.J. McBride, and S.M. Wolinsky. 1993. Detection of HIV-1 DNA and messenger RNA in individual cells by PCR-driven in situ hybridization and flow cytometry. *Science* **260:** 976.

Piatak, M., M.S. Saag, L.C. Yang, S.J. Clark, J.C. Kappes, K.-C. Luk, B.H. Hanh, G.M. Shaw, and J.D. Lifson. 1993. High levels of HIV-1 in plasma during all stages of infection determined by competitive PCR. *Science* **259:** 1749.

Posnett, D.N., S. Kabak, A.S. Hodtsev, E.A. Goldberg, and A. Asch. 1993a. TCR-Vβ subsets are not preferentially deleted in AIDS. *AIDS* **7:** 625.

Posnett, D.N., K. Mehta, S. Kabak, A.S. Hodtsev, A. Asch, E.A. Goldberg, J. Laurence, and P. Cameron. 1993b. HIV-1 DNA preferentially distributed in certain Vβ subsets. *FASEB J.* **150:** 179A.

Posnett, D.N., A. Gottlieb, J.B. Bussel, S.M. Friedman, N. Chiorazzi,

Y. Li, P. Szabo, N.R. Farid, and M.A. Robinson. 1988. T cell antigen receptors in autoimmunity. *J. Immunol.* **141:** 1963.

Salk, J., P.A. Bretscher, P.L. Salk, M. Clerici, and G.M. Shearer. 1993. A strategy for prophylactic vaccination against HIV. *Science* **260:** 1270.

Schnittman, S.M., M.C. Psallidopoulos, H.C. Lane, L. Thompson, M. Baseler, F. Massari, C.H. Fox, N.P. Salzman, and A.S. Fauci. 1989. The reservoir for HIV-1 in human peripheral blood is a T cell that maintains expression of CD4. *Science* **245:** 305.

Starcich, B.R., B.H. Hahn, G.M. Shaw, P.D. McNeely, S. Modrow, H. Wolf, E.S. Parks, W.P. Parks, S.F. Josephs, R.C. Gallo, and F. Wong-Staal. 1986. Identification and characterization of conserved and variable regions in the envelope gene of HTLVIII/LAV, the retrovirus of AIDS. *Cell* **45:** 637.

Waanders, G.A., A.N. Shakhov, W. Held, O. Karapetian, H. Acha-Orbea, and H.R. MacDonald. 1993. Peripheral T cell activation and deletion induced by transfer of lymphocyte subsets expressing endogenous or exogenous mouse mammary tumor virus. *J. Exp. Med.* **177:** 1359.

Wolinsky, S.M., C.M. Wike, B.T.M. Korber, C. Hutto, W.P. Parks, L.L. Rosenblum, K.J. Kunstman, M.R. Furtado, and J.L. Munoz. 1992. Selective transmission of human immunodeficiency virus type-1 variants from mothers to infants. *Science* **255:** 1134.

Index

αCRD3, 24
AIDS, 140, 147–150, 152, 171
  lack of preferential deletion of
    Vβ subsets in AIDS, 169–
    170
Anergy, 32, 109
Antigen-presenting cells, 125,
  164
  properties of RCS cells for Vβ16
    T-cell hybridomas, 99–100
Antisense S-oligonucleotides, 93
Apoptosis, 109, 148, 168–169

βCRD1, βCRD2, and βCRD3, 24
B cells, 47, 146
  activation, 144
  superantigen-induced, 36
B lymphoma cells, MTC-encoded
    expression in, 93–109

CD4⁺ T cells, 34–35, 93, 95, 127,
    129, 139, 144, 147–148,
    154–155, 169
CD8⁺ T cells, 95, 154
"Clonal deletion," 32, 59, 65–67,
    80–81
  influence of polymorphism of Vβ
    genes on, 67–68
COP wild mouse strain, 62–64,
    67

Enterotoxins, 139. See also
    specific enterotoxin
  staphylococcal, 2–3, 7
    SEA, 7–10, 12–20, 23–25, 139
    SEB, 7–8, 78, 80, 86, 148
  streptococcal, 7
    SPE-A and SPE-B, 10

env, 52–56, 154, 168
Epstein-Barr virus, 122, 140–
    141, 172, 174

Flow cytometric analysis, 145
Follicular cellular lymphomas
    (RSCs), 93
  RCS-Mtv, 93, 102, 105–108
Food poisoning. See Enterotoxins

gag, 52, 54, 144, 166, 170

Hemophilia, 171
Hepatitis B and C viruses, 171
HIV, 32
HIV-1, 140–141, 147–150, 152–
    156
  replication in T cells dependent
    on TCR Vβ expression,
    163–174
HVS, 140–141
Hydrocortisone, effect on
    superantigen-mediated
    neonatal deletion, 128
Hypervariable 4 (HV4), 26
  domain, 23
  loop, 24–25

Interleukin-2 (IL-2), 54, 98, 107,
    164
Interleukin-4 (IL-4), 107, 109
Interleukin-5 (IL-5), 107, 109

MAIDS, 140–141
  superantigens in the
    pathogenesis of MAIDS,
    144–145

Major histocompatibility complex (MHC) 1, 75, 85, 139, 149
  binding properties, 3–4, 9
  MHC class II, 8, 10, 25, 120, 154, 172
    binding site on SEA, 15, 23
    zinc and, 15–16, 20–23
    kinetic binding constant, 16–17
  molecule, 76
  polymorphism, 76
  -specific recognition, 88
  of Mls-1, 84–85
MAM, 122, 131, 133, 139
Mammary tumors, 45, 48. *See also* Mouse mammary tumor virus
Minor lymphocyte stimulating (Mls) antigens, 1, 7, 59, 64, 127, 131
Mls-1, 76, 78, 84–85
mls, 140, 142
Mouse mammary tumor virus (MMTV), 2, 26, 76, 117, 141, 152, 155, 163, 167
  analogies between life cycle of MMTV and MAIDS, 144–145
  env and, 52–56
  -induced tumorigenesis
    MMTV *env* and *sag* stimulation of T cells in vivo, 52–56
    sag and, 48–50
  life cycle, 38–40
  -LTR, 93, 100–102
  mechanism for transmission, 48
  MMTV(SW), 35–37
  sag-mediated deletions, 148
  superantigen proteins, 47–48
  superantigens expressed by MMTV
    anti-*orf* monoclonal antibodies, 37–38
    infectious MMTVs, 34–37
    orf, 32–33
  TCR Vβ in wild mice and, 64–65
Mtv-8, 93

Natural populations, TCR Vβ in wild mice, 60
nef, 34, 154, 174
"Negative selection," 127
NJ101, B-cell lymphoma, 93, 97, 102
N protein of rabies virus, 122, 133
  binding to human MHC class II molecules, 120–122
  physical properties, 118–119
Nucleocapsid (NC) protein of rabies virus, 117–134, 139, 145
  binding to MHC class II molecules, 120–122
  physical properties, 118–119
Nude mice, rabies virus infection in, 145

Open reading frame, 163
orf, 32, 103
  anti-*orf* monoclonal antibodies, 37–38
  superantigens encoded by MMTV *orf*, 32–33

Peyer's patches, 39
pol, 52, 54
Polymerase chain reaction, 148, 150–151, 166, 169, 171
Proviruses, 32, 45, 47

Rabies virus (RV)
  -associated superantigen activity, 146
  nucleocapsid, 141
  superantigenicity in humans and mice, 117–134
  superantigens in RV infection, 145–147
Retrovirus, MMTV as retrovirus. *See* Mouse mammary tumor virus
"Reversed immunological surveillance," 94

sag, 48–52, 139–140, 148, 152
SEA, 7–8, 18
  functional binding sites, 7–25
  zinc-binding site, 19–21
SEB, 7–8
SEC1–3, 8, 10
SED, 8, 18, 25
SEE, 8, 10–12, 18, 25, 139, 166
  structure of SEA/SEE hybrids,
    13
SIV, 141
SJL mice, 63–64, 66–67, 146
  superantigen in lymphoma-host
    T-cell interaction in, 93–
    109
Superantigens (sAgs), 75. *See
    also specific superantigen*
  brief history, 1–4
  enterotoxins as sAgs, 133. *See
    also* Enterotoxins
  exogenous virus sAgs, 117
  function, 3–4
  in HIV-1 infection and AIDS,
    147–150, 152–154
  the pathogenesis of viral dis-
    eases and, 139–156
  structure of endogenous sAgs,
    68
  T-cell recognition
    role of MHC molecules and,
      81–84
    role of non-Vβ TCR elements
      and, 75–81
  viruses encoding v-sAgs, 141

T cells, 36, 47, 59, 81, 168
  activation, 139, 144, 147
  and HIV-1, 155
  CD4+, 34–35, 93
  hybridomas, 93
  Mls-reactive T cells, 1
  receptor (TCR), 2, 7, 31, 54, 75,
    81, 139, 148, 163
  α-chain elements, 77–80
  β-chain, 15, 61, 139, 148
  plate binding assay, 15
  proteins, 9–10. *See also
    specific protein*

binding properties, 3
binding site, 12–15
  on SEA, 23
  Jα, 77, 85
  single chain, 15
  TCR/superantigen interac-
    tions, 2–4
  Vα, 77–80, 93, 149
  Vβ, 8–9, 23–24, 31, 34, 75,
    117, 122, 164
  -binding site, 15
  contact residues, 14
  -deleting elements, 62
  determinants, 155
  of SEA and SEE, 12
  -determining residues, 14
  domains, 2
  clonal deletions in wild mice,
    59–69
  HIV-1 replication dependent
    on Vβ expression, 163–174
  non-Vβ elements, 76–80
  repertoire, 12, 142, 148–152
  -specific monoclonal
    antibodies, 163–164
  Vβ2 T cells, 66, 128
  Vβ6 and 7 T cells in BALB/c
    mice, 126, 130–131, 133–
    134
  Vβ8 T cells in humans, 123,
    125, 132, 170
  Vβ12 T cells, 170–171, 173
  Vβ14 T cells, 142
  Vβ16 T cells, 93, 96–98, 106,
    150

RCS-responsive T cells, func-
    tional properties, 95–96
  recognition of sAgs, 84–89
  role of MHC molecule, 81–84
  role for non-Vβ elements, 76–
    80
  stimulation and role of RCS-
    specific MMTV-LTR ORF
    products, 105–106
  tolerance, influence of TCR α
    chain, 80–81
TIIIB, 166–167

TSST, 10–11
TSST-1, 8, 131, 133, 139, 166
Toxic shock syndrome, 8–10

Vα, 77–80, 93
Vβ, 8–9, 23–24, 31, 34, 75, 117,
    122
  -binding site, 15
  contact residues, 14
  -deleting elements, 62
  determinants of SEA and SEE,
    12
  -determining residues, 14
  domains, 2
    clonal deletions in wild mice,
    59–69
  non-Vβ elements, 76–80
  repertoire, 12
Vβ2 T cells, 66, 128

Vβ6 and 7 T cells in BALB/c
    mice, 126, 130–131, 133–
    134
Vβ8 T cells in humans, 123, 125,
    132
Vβ12 T cells, 170–171, 173
Vβ14 T cells, 142
Vβ16 T cells, 93, 96–98, 106, 150

WLA wild mouse strain, 62–64

Zinc, 19, 23–25
  binding, 15–16
    and enterotoxins, 20–21, 23
  -binding motif, 20
  bridge with MHC class II
    residue, 22–23
  coordination, 20
  ^{65}Zn binding, 20, 22